DEMENTIA CARE MAPPING

DEMENTIA CARE MAPPING

APPLICATIONS
ACROSS CULTURES

edited by

Anthea Innes, M.Sc., Ph.D.
University of Stirling
Scotland

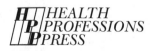

HEALTH PROFESSIONS PRESS

Baltimore • London • Winnipeg • Sydney

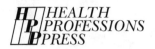

Health Professions Press, Inc.
Post Office Box 10624
Baltimore, Maryland 21285-0624

www.healthpropress.com

Typeset by Auburn Associates, Inc., Baltimore, Maryland.
Manufactured in the United States of America by
Versa Press, East Peoria, Illinois.

Far-right cover photograph by Terry Joseph Sam. All other cover photographs by
Bill Richert.

The stories in this book are based on the authors' experiences. In some cases, names and
other identifying information have been changed to protect individuals' identities. Other
vignettes are composite accounts that do not represent the lives or experiences of specific
individuals, and no implications should be inferred.

Library of Congress Cataloging-in-Publication Data

Dementia care mapping : applications across cultures / edited by Anthea Innes.
    p.   cm.
Includes bibliographical references and index.
ISBN 1-878812-84-X
    1. Dementia—Patients—Care—Evaluation.   2. Dementia—Patients—Care—
Cross-cultural studies.   I. Innes, Anthea.
    RC521.D4537 2002 2003
    362.1'9683—dc21

                           2002027616

British Library Cataloguing in Publication data are available from the British Library.

CONTENTS

ABOUT THE EDITOR

Anthea Innes, M.Sc., Ph.D., became involved in the teaching, development, and use of Dementia Care Mapping (DCM) for research purposes while she worked at the Bradford Dementia Group from 1997 to 2001. She became interested in the cultural applications of DCM during her involvement in setting up a DCM strategic partnership with the Heather Hill Hospital in Chardon, Ohio.

Dr. Innes, an Approved Dementia Care Mapping Evaluator and Trainer, works at the Centre for Social Research on Dementia at the University of Stirling, Scotland. Her post involves the development of social gerontological research, with a specific emphasis on dementia. Her primary research interest is dementia and dementia care; within this broad area, her work has focused on the experiences of people with dementia and of informal caregivers and paid care workers. She is particularly interested in groups that are marginalized in relation to dementia and dementia care. To date, this concern has centered on minority ethnic groups, unqualified care staff, and dementia in rural areas. Dr. Innes also is interested in the development and use of methods to elicit the views of people with dementia and in process issues involved in the conduct of research.

Dr. Innes wrote *Training and Development for Dementia Care Workers* (Jessica Kingsley Publishers, 1999). With Karen Hatfield, she co-edited *Healing Arts Therapies and Person-Centred Dementia Care* (Jessica Kingsley Publishers, 2001). In addition, she has authored or co-authored articles appearing in journals such as *Ageing and Mental Health* and *Education and Ageing*.

CONTRIBUTORS

Dawn Brooker, Ph.D.,
C. Psychol. (Clin.)
Strategic Lead Dementia Care
  Mapping
Approved Dementia Care Mapping
  Evaluator and Trainer
Bradford Dementia Group
School of Health Studies
University of Bradford
Unity Building
25 Trinity Road
Bradford BD5 0BB
England

Andrea Capstick, B.A. (Hons.)
Approved Dementia Care Mapping
  Evaluator and Trainer
Lecturer in Dementia Studies
Bradford Dementia Group
School of Health Studies
University of Bradford
Unity Building
25 Trinity Road
Bradford BD5 0BB
England

Lisa Heller, S.R.N.
  (State Registered Nurse)
Approved Dementia Care Mapping
  Evaluator and Trainer
Dementia Care Mapping Service
Sheffield Community National
  Health Service Trust
Services for Older People and
  Rehabilitation
The Longley Centre
Norwood Grange Drive
Sheffield S5 7JT
England

Cordelia Man-yuk Kwok,
  master's degree in health
  service management
Nurse Specialist (Psychogeriatric),
  diploma in psychiatric nursing
Approved Dementia Care Mapping
  Evaluator
Kwai Chung Hospital
3-15 Kwai Chung Hospital Road, NT
Hong Kong, SAR
China

Carolyn Lechner, M.S.S.A., L.S.W.
Approved Dementia Care Mapping
  Evaluator and Trainer
Heather Hill Hospital
12340 Bass Lake Road
Chardon, OH 44024
United States of America

Tracey Lintern, Ph.D.
Dementia Services Development
  Centre Wales
Neuadd Ardudwy
University of Wales–Bangor
Normal Site, Holyhead Road
Bangor LL57 2PX
Wales

Virgina Moore, Bachelor of
  Applied Science, O.T.,
  Diploma of O.T., O.T.R.
Churchill Fellow
Approved Dementia Care Mapping
  Evaluator and Trainer
Manager Specialist Services
Brightwater Care Group
Post Office Box 762
Osbourne Park, WA 6016
Australia

Christian Müller-Hergl,
  Dipl. Theol., B.Phil.,
  Registered Geriatric Nurse
Approved Dementia Care Mapping
  Evaluator and Trainer
Meinwerk-Institut
Giersmauer 35
33098 Paderborn
Germany

Michelle Persaud, R.N.M.H.
  (Registered Nurse Mental
  Handicap), M.A.
Approved Dementia Care Mapping
  Evaluator
Nurse Consultant (Dual Diagnosis)
Derbyshire Mental Health Services
  Trust
Aston Hall Hospital
Aston-on-Trent, Derbyshire
  DE72 2AL
England

Maria Scurfield-Walton, B.S.,
  Dip. Nursing, R.M.N.
Approved Dementia Care Mapping
  Evaluator and Trainer
Practice Development Nurse
South of Tyne and Wearside
  National Health Service Trust
Cherry Knowle Hospital
Ryhope, Sunderland
Tyne and Wear SR2 0NB
England

Bob Woods, M.A., M.Sc.,
  C. Psychol., F.B.Ps.S.
Professor
Co-Director
Dementia Services Development
  Centre Wales
Neuadd Ardudwy
University of Wales–Bangor
Normal Site, Holyhead Road
Bangor LL57 2PX
Wales

TRAINING PROGRAM CONTACTS

Please contact the following individuals for further information on Dementia Care Mapping (DCM) training and evaluations.

**General inquiries
and United Kingdom**
Dawn Brooker
Strategic Lead Dementia Care
  Mapping
Approved Dementia Care Mapping
  Evaluator and Trainer
Bradford Dementia Group
School of Health Studies
University of Bradford
Unity Building
25 Trinity Road
Bradford BD5 0BB
England
Telephone: +44 (0) 1274 233996
Fax: +44 (0) 1274 236395
E-mail: d.j.brooker@bradford.ac.uk

Australia
Virginia Moore
Churchill Fellow
Approved Dementia Care Mapping
  Evaluator and Trainer
Manager Specialist Services
Brightwater Care Group
Post Office Box 762
Osbourne Park, WA 6016
Australia
Telephone: +61 (08) 9444 2311
Fax: +61 (08) 9444 2355
E-mail: virginia@brightwater.asn.au

Denmark
Eva Bonde Nielsen
Approved Dementia Care Mapping
  Evaluator and Trainer
Director
Danish National Institute
  for Elderly Education (DANIEE)
Degnemose Alle 83
DK-2700 Bronshoj
Denmark
Telephone: +45 3860 6091
E-mail: ebn@daniae.dk

Germany
Christian Müller-Hergl
Approved Dementia Care Mapping
  Evaluator and Trainer
Meinwerk-Institut
Giersmauer 35
33098 Paderborn
Germany
Telephone: +49 5251 2908 30
Fax: +49 5251 2908 68
E-mail: herglboecklin27@aol.com

United States of America
Roseann Kasayka
Approved Dementia Care Mapping
  Evaluator and Trainer
Heather Hill Hospital
Health and Care Center
12340 Bass Lake Road
Chardon, OH 44024
United States of America
Telephone: +1 (440) 279-2409
Fax: +1 (440) 285-7743
E-mail: rkasayka@heatherhill.org

FOREWORD

Since the late 1970s, it has been increasingly recognized that people with dementia are experiencing a disease process (often Alzheimer's disease) and not "normal aging." With this recognition has come the growth of the dementia care field. Care worker practice and health care research have yielded a wealth of knowledge and approaches that can support the personhood of individuals with dementia. Yet, research and best care practices are just starting to be visible in the real-world settings where people with dementia live and receive care.

Enter Dementia Care Mapping (DCM). The work of Kitwood and Bredin had its inception in the late 1980s and shifted the discussion about the goals of specialized dementia care. DCM is one of the first methods to focus on the outcomes of dementia care. DCM does for dementia care what outcomes measurement has done for much of health care and social services. It asks a few fundamental questions: What are good outcomes of dementia care? If the needs of a person with dementia are being met, what does that look like? Can it be measured? Can that measurement be used to evaluate current care and to individualize care plans to support the person's well-being?

DCM has great appeal to those who care deeply about people with dementia. The method has generated feelings of "at last!" to those of us who want so desperately for dementia care to do justice for those who have dementia. *Dementia Care Mapping: Applications Across Cultures* explores the early DCM work that has been conducted across care settings and across several cultures. The time for this discussion is now, and this book explores the early successes of DCM as well as its limitations.

Ultimately, *Dementia Care Mapping: Applications Across Cultures* reviews DCM and its current place in the field of dementia care and outcomes measurement. It raises as many questions as answers about the effectiveness and usability of DCM as a person-centered evaluator of dementia care. Nonetheless, these discussions are well begun, as DCM's place within the field of dementia care is being explored and debated.

Anna Ortigara, R.N., M.S.
Vice President of Program Development
Life Services Network
Hinsdale, Illinois

INTRODUCTION

ANTHEA INNES

Since the 1990s, Dementia Care Mapping (DCM) has grown from small be-
ginnings into an internationally recognized method to evaluate dementia care.
What attracts individuals to the DCM method? DCM's rise in popularity may
in part be attributed to the general increase of interest in dementia and
dementia care and to a desire within health care for outcome measures. DCM
has been further endorsed by government reports (e.g., Audit Commission,
2000) that recommend it as a tool for evaluating dementia care. A large number of individuals have participated in DCM training within the United
Kingdom, where it was developed, and in other countries (Innes, Capstick, &
Surr, 2000). Those who have received training include social workers, nurses,
care assistants, psychologists, physicians, and researchers, suggesting a widespread attraction to this method.

OVERVIEW OF THE DEMENTIA CARE MAPPING METHOD

DCM was designed in the late 1980s in response to a service provider's request
for an evaluation of its dementia care services (Kitwood & Bredin, 1992). The
method has undergone many developments since its inception, and the training manual, currently in its seventh edition (Bradford Dementia Group,
1997), reflects the suggestions of experienced users (called *mappers*). DCM is a
tool that provides a way to measure the extent to which the person-centered

1

approach to care (Kitwood, 1997) is a reality for people with dementia who live in formal care settings. The DCM method also offers an assessment of the care process and outcomes for people with dementia.

DCM highlights not only areas of care practice that need improvement but also areas of staff strength to build on and develop. The mapper gathers detailed information about the care setting as a whole and about each person with dementia in that setting. Although the detailed observation process is time consuming and can, by design, only take place in public areas, DCM tells us much about *the person with dementia's experience* of care provision in formal care settings because the care setting is evaluated as thoroughly as possible from the point of view of each person receiving care. This focus on the person with dementia's experience was and is perhaps the most innovative aspect of DCM. Observing from this viewpoint is important given concerns about the reliability of self-report by people with dementia (Rabins & Kasper, 1997) and the absence of alternative, fully developed, and evaluated methods.

CONDUCTING A DEMENTIA CARE MAPPING EVALUATION

A full DCM evaluation occurs for 6 consecutive hours on 2 days—for example, 2 P.M.–8 P.M. on the first day and 8 A.M.–2 P.M. on the second day—to ensure that the whole care day is observed. The 6-hour observation period is divided into 5-minute intervals, called *time frames*. Continuous time sampling is used to record data. If more than two mappers are evaluating the care setting, then a 1-hour reliability test is conducted prior to the evaluation to enhance the reliability and validity of the observations. One mapper can observe 5–10 participants. The decision to include an individual in the evaluation depends on the person having a diagnosis of dementia, his or her presence in public areas on the days of the evaluation, and his or her consent.

Four coding frames are used to record information. The first coding frame, Behaviour Category Coding (BCC), is used to record the behavior in which each person with dementia is engaged. For each 5-minute observation period, the mapper selects the most appropriate Behaviour Category from a list of 24 different types of behaviors, ranging from participating in games to sleeping (see Table 1).

The second coding frame captures the Well- or Ill-Being (WIB) of each person during each 5-minute observation period. WIB values range from −5 to +5 and indicate the extent to which an individual is in a state of well- or ill-being in each 5-minute time frame (see Table 2). The observer follows guidelines in the DCM manual (Bradford Dementia Group, 1997) to record a

Table 1. Behaviour Category Coding (BCC)

Code	Memory cue	General description of category
A	Articulation	Interacting verbally or otherwise
B	Borderline	Being socially involved, but passively
C	Cool	Being socially uninvolved, withdrawn
D	Distress	Unattended distress
E	Expression	Engaging in an expressive or creative activity
F	Food	Eating, drinking
G	Games	Participating in a game
H	Handicraft	Participating in a craft activity
I	Intellectual	Activity prioritizing the use of intellectual abilities
J	Joints	Participating in exercise or physical games
K	Kum and go	Independent walking, standing, or moving in a wheelchair
L	Labour	Performing work or a work-like activity
M	Media	Engaging with media
N	Nod, land of	Sleeping, dozing
O	Own care	Independently engaging in self-care
P	Physical care	Receiving practical, physical, or personal care
R	Religion	Participating in a religious activity
S	Sex	Engaging in an activity related to explicit sexual expression
T	Timalation	Directly engaging the senses
U	Unresponded to	Communicating without receiving a response
W	Withstanding	Engaging in repetitive self-stimulation
X	X-cretion	Episodes related to excretion
Y	Yourself	Talking to oneself or an imagined person, hallucinating
Z	Zero option	Engaging in behaviors that do not fit in an existing category

From Bradford Dementia Group. (1997). *Evaluating dementia care: The DCM method* (7th ed., pp. 23–24). Bradford, England: University of Bradford; adapted by permission.

WIB value. This value indicates the observer's judgment of the quality of the interaction or quality of life as experienced by the person with dementia. These figures are aggregated to 1) find the overall WIB score for the group and for each individual and 2) provide an overall profile of the proportion of time that the group and the individuals observed spent in each level of well- or ill-being.

A third coding frame is used to record instances in which residents are put down in some way. These are selected from Kitwood's (1997) 17 examples of malignant social psychology, known in DCM terms as Personal Detractions (PDs). Examples of PDs include objectification (treating the person as though he or she were an object), infantilization (treating the person as though he or she were a child), and ignoring (talking over the person or disregarding his or

Table 2. Well-Being and Ill-Being (WIB) value coding

WIB value code	General description of code
+5	Exceptional well-being: it is hard to envision anything better; very high levels of engagement, self-expression, and social interaction
+3	Considerable well-being (e.g., in engagement, interaction, and initiation of social contact)
+1	Adequate coping with the present situation: some contact with others; no observed signs of ill-being
−1	Slight ill-being (e.g., boredom, restlessness, frustration)
−3	Considerable ill-being (e.g., sadness, fear, sustained anger, moving deeper into apathy and withdrawal, continued neglect for longer than a half an hour)
−5	Obvious ill-being: extreme apathy or withdrawal, rage, grief or despair, continued neglect for longer than an hour

From Bradford Dementia Group. (1997). *Evaluating dementia care: The DCM method* (7th ed., pp. 23–24). Bradford, England: University of Bradford; adapted by permission.

her ability to communicate). The severity level of instances in which PDs occur is also recorded, ranging from mild and moderate to severe and very severe.

A fourth, less-structured coding frame is used to record positive events. Instances in which the well-being of a person with dementia is enhanced are used to formulate a Positive Event Record (PER). Examples include staff showing sensitivity and skill or validating an individual's feelings. This coding frame is the least developed of the four; however, it offers a way to capture many aspects of what has been coined as *positive person work* (Kitwood, 1997). This is when care staff display empathy, sensitivity, or skill in their practice— for example, the feelings of the person with dementia are acknowledged and validated. In addition, when applied to specific therapies such as dance, music, and art (Innes & Hatfield, 2001), it has much to offer the therapist or practitioner seeking to evaluate the effectiveness and impact of an activity for a person with dementia.

THE PROCESS OF A DEMENTIA CARE MAPPING EVALUATION

The intention of using DCM developmentally (e.g., to develop care practice over time) is to empower staff in their work. Empowerment can be attained through operationalizing one of the method's guiding principles: openness (Bradford Dementia Group, 1997). Table 3 details a process to achieve openness throughout a DCM evaluation. In this process, the mapper clearly explains the purpose of the observation, or map, to all care staff; shares data with the whole staff group; and helps the staff group to develop action plans.

Table 3. Process of using mapping to achieve openness

Phase	Purpose
1. Set up and plan the map	Meet with those commissioning the evaluation and/or those with the power and responsibility to act or make the decision not to act on findings.
	Gain insights into the potential possibilities of and obstacles to action.
2. Brief staff	Give the mappers an opportunity to meet the staff in the care setting.
	Introduce the Dementia Care Mapping (DCM) method to staff.
	Answer any staff queries.
3. Conduct mapping	Make introductions to the client and staff group.
	Obtain informal consent from each participant (i.e., person with dementia to be observed).
	Be prepared to show the data sheets to the staff and participants.
	Answer any queries from the staff or participants.
	Help out if asked by staff member or participant.
	Intervene if necessary to avoid problems (e.g., a resident falling).
4. Conduct feedback sessions	Give all staff access to the data.
	Obtain staff feedback on the data.
5. Plan for the future	Encourage staff to develop their practice.
	Plan a second evaluation.
	Develop a realistic action plan.

Source: Innes (2000).

COMPARISION OF CULTURAL FACTORS IN APPLYING DEMENTIA CARE MAPPING

The idea for this book, which reflects and comments on the use of DCM in a variety of contexts or cultures, arose from my own DCM work in a number of care settings in the United Kingdom. Observing, or mapping, a range of settings highlighted the differences and similarities in using the DCM method within different cultures of care. While working at Bradford Dementia Group in England between 1997 and 2001, I helped teach the DCM method. This led to my interest in participants' use of the method in other parts of the world—namely the United States of America, Australia, Germany, Denmark, and Hong Kong—with different cultural values and different economic, political, and welfare systems. My interest further developed while working with Carolyn Lechner, a colleague from Heather Hill Hospital in Chardon,

Ohio. Carolyn Lechner and I began to engage in a comparative analysis of U.K. and U.S. DCM data sets. At the 2000 World Alzheimer Congress in Washington, D.C., the idea developed that a comparison of cultural factors in applying DCM would make a useful book.

OVERVIEW OF THIS BOOK

Dementia Care Mapping: Applications Across Cultures comprises four sections. Section I discusses broad issues relating to the use of the DCM method. Andrea Capstick, one of the longest-serving members of Bradford Dementia Group, has played key roles in the development of courses that teach others how to use DCM and in the application of person-centered care principles. In Chapter 1, she provides an overview of the theoretical basis of DCM. Issues of reliability and validity often perplex DCM users, both those using DCM for research purposes and those trying to convince service providers and commissioners of the method's value. These issues are examined in Chapter 2 by Bob Woods and Tracey Lintern, whose work has involved assessing the validity of DCM. Lisa Heller has used DCM in both health and social care settings. In Chapter 3, she discusses the notion of *culture of care,* raising issues worthy of consideration by any DCM user whose aim is to influence and improve care practice.

Section II develops this point by considering the uses of DCM to improve care practice. Christian Müller-Hergl was one of the first people to use DCM outside of the United Kingdom. In Chapter 4, he discusses the method's potential to improve care practice and highlights potential difficulties in providing an institution with feedback that is based on its performance as indicated by DCM data. DCM data can also be used to improve care directly for those observed. In Chapter 5, I provide a practical example of using DCM data to improve care for individuals with dementia and discuss the potential use of DCM data to develop care plans. Before DCM can be implemented to improve care, however, staff development opportunities may be required. Maria Scurfield-Walton highlights this point in Chapter 6. She also presents the concept of using DCM itself as a vehicle to identify further staff development needs, thereby improving staff skills, increasing staff confidence levels, and enabling care workers to develop and improve their care practice.

Section III considers policy issues that are pertinent to implementing DCM in different countries. Virginia Moore has sought to implement DCM in Australia, where the care system and policies—and, thus, the policy context—are different from those of the United Kingdom. In Chapter 7, she highlights these matters and discusses the use of DCM to influence organizational policy—a key step to the effective use of DCM at the microcare level. DCM can contradict the "good sense" of traditional medical models of care (see Chapter 1), and Cordelia Man-yuk Kwok considers this issue in Chapter 8 within the context of Hong Kong's distinctive culture, medical traditions, and language. Her chapter shows that DCM can be compatible with traditional medical traditions, as it gives care providers opportunities to provide a higher quality of care service. Carolyn Lechner brings together policy issues in Chapter 9. Anyone seeking to use DCM would be wise to consider her discussion of social, political, and economic factors that influence the climate of care provision.

Section IV considers future uses of DCM. Michelle Persaud is one of the few research practitioners who has examined using DCM with people with cognitive disabilities. In Chapter 10, she discusses the strengths and limitations of using DCM to observe an alternative client group as well as a possible future in using DCM to evaluate care for a number of other groups. A new edition of the DCM manual is planned for 2004, so Chapter 10 develops the theme of DCM's future uses. In Chapter 11, Dawn Brooker discusses the rationale for such uses and possible variations of the method to suit alternative purposes. *Dementia Care Mapping: Applications Across Cultures* concludes with a critical consideration of the future popularity and use of the DCM method.

This book cannot claim to offer definitive answers about how to improve care practice through the use of DCM. It is hoped that the readers of this book, whether they are new to the method or experienced mappers, will gain insights into the use of DCM within different care settings and in different countries. Those currently using the method may find ideas to become more effective (i.e., to improve care) in their use of the method within a care setting. For those who are new to the DCM method, it is envisaged that this book provides an overview of the method and its theoretical origins (Section I) while highlighting the ways that DCM can be used to improve care practice (Section II) in a variety of settings and in countries with different cultures (Sections III and IV). *Dementia Care Mapping: Applications Across Cultures* aims therefore to make a contribution to the understanding of the application of DCM in different cultures and to the potential ways in which DCM can be used to improve the lives of people with dementia.

REFERENCES

Audit Commission. (2000). *Forget me not: Mental health services for older people.* London: Author.
Bradford Dementia Group. (1997). *Evaluating dementia care: The DCM method* (7th ed.). Bradford, England: University of Bradford.

Innes, A. (2000). Dementia care mapping. In H. Staber, M. Cofone, D.V. Saarlouis, & L. Saarlouis (Eds.), *Innovativer umgang mit dementen: Strategien, konzepte und einrichtungen in Europa* (pp. 117–121). Germany: Demenz-Verein Sarlouis eV.

Innes, A., Capstick, A., & Surr, C. (2000). Mapping out the framework. *Journal of Dementia Care, 8*(2), 20–21.

Innes, A., & Hatfield, K. (Eds.). (2001). *Healing arts therapies and person-centred dementia care*. London: Jessica Kingsley Publishers.

Kitwood, T. (1997). *Dementia reconsidered: The person comes first*. Buckingham, England: Open University Press.

Kitwood, T., & Bredin, K. (1992). *The Dementia Care Mapping method*. Bradford, England: University of Bradford.

Rabins, P.V., & Kasper, J.D. (1997). Measuring quality of life in dementia: Conceptual and practical issues. *Alzheimer's Disease and Associated Disorders, 11*(6), 100–104.

I

THE DEMENTIA
CARE MAPPING
METHOD

1

THE THEORETICAL ORIGINS OF DEMENTIA CARE MAPPING

ANDREA CAPSTICK

> *Maps do transcribe*
> *physical space.*
> *They also in a sense*
> *inscribe it, with names,*
> *boundary lines and*
> *even . . . a perspective*
> *from which to view it.*
> *—Anthony Fothergill*
> *(1989)*

Cartography—the science of map making—has often involved charting unknown territory. In one sense, making maps can be an entirely helpful occupation. Maps provide travelers with information that helps them get from their current location to their destination. Dementia Care Mapping (DCM) can be viewed in this way—as a route that helps care workers improve the quality of care for people who have dementia.

In another sense, as the literature on colonialism and imperialism clearly demonstrates, map making can be a problematic pursuit. The territory in question is not unknown to those who inhabit it; it is only unknown to the map makers, whose observations and measurements may be based on different cultural imperatives and perspectives. Historically, the mapping of territories was often linked with dispossession and alienation. This risk also exists for DCM if those who practice it are not entirely clear about the value base from which they are operating. The origins of DCM in the bodies of psychological theory and ethical frameworks embraced by Tom Kitwood, DCM's founder, are thus worthy of detailed consideration. They provide the subject matter for this chapter.

Although not without its critics, DCM is now a popular and well-established method for evaluating quality of life (QOL) for people with dementia. DCM is a method for observing and coding the current quality of care for people with dementia in group care settings (Bradford Dementia Group, 1997). It provides a means of gathering data about the range of activities in which clients are involved and about their apparent emotional well-being. These data suggest improvements that can be made in planning future care. In this sense, DCM may provide a useful "map" to inform the development of care practice.

In England, the Audit Commission (2000) recommended DCM as a means of monitoring the quality of dementia care services. DCM's influence is spreading rapidly across the globe. As of 2002, mappers comprise ten nationalities, and DCM courses are available on three continents. In many ways, this is a remarkable success story for a method that was developed little more than 10 years ago. It is even more notable in view of the somewhat radical theoretical and philosophical underpinnings of DCM. It begins to verge on the extraordinary when one considers that many of the key terms used in a DCM evaluation (e.g., *QOL, quality of care, well-being, ill-being*) have never been fully defined or operationalized and that its measures have not been standardized for research purposes.

There is evidently something very powerful about DCM. It has the ability to engage the interest and imagination of care practitioners. It is beginning to speak in a universal language to those who are committed to the improvement of dementia care. DCM, at its best, has the potential to provide striking insights into both the current quality of dementia care provision and into what may be achieved in this field. If it is not handled carefully, however, DCM has the potential to undermine and to negate the efforts of frontline workers. This chapter explores how both the strengths and limitations of DCM in its current form can be traced back to its theoretical origins.

TENDER-HEARTED THEORY, TOUGH-MINDED METHOD

Neither its enthusiasts nor its critics have engaged much with DCM at a theoretical level, which has led to a number of misunderstandings and occasional abuses. If there is to be an informed debate about the value of DCM and its future role in developing dementia care practice across cultures, then it is important to avoid an unbridgeable theory–practice divide. DCM practiced solely as a method, without reference to an underlying philosophy of care, could easily degenerate into a mere measurement-for-measurement's sake assessment tool.

A common misunderstanding is confusing the DCM method with the person-centered approach to dementia care. Much of DCM's popularity arises from its association with the person-centered approach, and it is still not unusual for the two terms to be confused with each other. It is often assumed that training staff in DCM automatically leads to the implementation of person-centered care. As many organizations are beginning to discover, however, DCM is more likely to reveal serious deficiencies in existing care provision than to provide a magical quick fix. Moreover, although DCM can be used to evaluate the extent to which person-centered care is being implemented, it can be argued that it is not an inherently person-centered or humanistic method. DCM can and has been used in ways that are inconsistent with its stated aim of improving the QOL for those with dementia (e.g., to supervise individual members of staff, to make decisions about the placement of individuals whom staff find troublesome).

The strongest claim to person centeredness in the DCM method itself is that observers take the standpoint of the person with dementia and make a subjective assessment of what the person is experiencing. The observer codes each 5-minute time frame according to the DCM manual's scale of Well- and Ill-Being (WIB) values (see Table 2 in the Introduction). In the DCM manual Kitwood pointed out,

> Doing this involves a great deal more than simple observation. It requires the faculty known as empathy: being able to put oneself, imaginatively, into the place of another person, and sense what life may be like from within that person's frame of reference. (Bradford Dementia Group, 1997, p. 5)

The concept of empathy, or *empathic awareness,* is one drawn from Rogerian humanistic theory and does indeed lie at the heart of person-centered approaches to care. Empathic awareness, however, is normally taken to require sustained personal interaction and a knowledge of the individual's circumstances. It can be difficult to gain this degree of empathy merely by observing from a distance.

States of well-being are relatively easy to identify. It is reasonable to assume that a person with dementia displaying affection, humor, and enjoyment or initiating contact with others is evidence of well-being. These signs are consistent in all human beings across cultures. Such signs may not, however, be directly related to quality of care, particularly in those who are relatively new to a care setting. Signs of ill-being are more difficult to identify by observation and are more culturally relative. This is particularly true of the Behaviour Category Code *C* (Cool—socially uninvolved; see Table 1 in the Introduction for a complete list of codes). According to DCM, this state of social disengagement is never consistent with well-being, and it cannot be coded together with a positive WIB value. Although apathy and withdrawal are rightly viewed as indicators of ill-being in DCM, a number of critics have pointed out that it is impossible to assess someone's inner state when he or she is engaged in this form of activity (or inactivity). What appears to be social withdrawal may be a pleasant state of reverie, daydreaming, or even something akin to meditation. It seems likely that many older people will spend part of their time in quiet reflection, regardless of environment. In other cases, it may well be that a participant is being allowed to drift into a virtually catatonic state through lack of sensory stimulation. DCM observers cannot, however, rely on empathy to distinguish between the two states. A further issue here is that DCM is perhaps biased toward a level of activity and occupation typical of Western industrialized societies rather than of societies with a less materialistic or achievement-oriented way of life.

As an observational method, DCM would initially tend to be classified as qualitative. However, the data-processing operations carried out on this qualitative data are in keeping with those same quantitative traditions of scientific inquiry from which Kitwood often sought to distance himself. DCM is a peculiar harnessing together of tender-hearted theory and tough-minded method. In practice, this can raise problems: Those attracted to the person-centered approach for its warmth and empathy often find uninteresting the intensive data processing and analysis of DCM and, therefore, do not always master the techniques sufficiently to conduct DCM accurately. At the same time, those attracted to DCM for its ability to provide hard data about quality of care may have little interest in practice development.

In some ways, then, it appears that there is a fundamental lack of fit between the theory and the method of DCM. To explore this concept further, the following section considers the various strands of theory that informed Kitwood's early work in the field of dementia care, as well as his initial work to develop DCM.

Dementia Care Mapping's
Challenge to the Standard Paradigm

Kitwood and Bredin began developing DCM in the late 1980s (see Kitwood & Bredin, 1992a). The extent to which this development was driven initially by the person-centered approach is not as clear as might be imagined, as this approach is not a strong theme in Kitwood's published work of the period.

A useful starting point for uncovering the theoretical background to DCM is the original research proposal to the Leverhulme Trust (Kitwood, 1991). Clearly, some developmental work had been done by the time the proposal was made. In addition, a feasibility study had been carried out as part of a project then in progress with Bradford Health Authority to evaluate its "day care provision" (sic) for people with dementia. (Although day care facilities have the specific function of providing activities and social interaction, DCM is now promoted as a means of evaluating QOL in all group care settings, including facilities and hospital wards, which do not have the same purpose as day care. Care settings of this nature will tend to evaluate poorly by comparison with the day care facilities for which DCM was originally intended.)

Kitwood's proposal to Leverhulme cites his "five main publications related to dementia" and clearly states that his "latest book sets out a psychological basis for the ethic of caregiving that underlies this proposal" (1991, p. 4). The book in question was the newly published *Concern for Others: A New Psychology of Conscience and Morality* (Kitwood, 1990a). This book makes only passing reference to dementia and is rarely cited among Kitwood's publications. Yet, it provides interesting insights into his theoretical concerns and affiliations during the period when DCM was under development. The book's dominant themes are moral development, moral responsibility, and the re-framing of psychology as a "moral science of action" rather than taking the traditional view of the discipline as the "science of behavior." The book suggests that the process of individual psychotherapy provides a useful model for a more morally integrated society. At the time, Kitwood was a lecturer in social psychology in the Faculty of Social Sciences at the University of Bradford in England. The Faculty's Directory of Expertise for 1991 (McLaren, Mellors, & Radtke, 1991) reiterated this emphasis, listing his research interests as

1. Senile dementia: social/biographical aspects in progress of illness; quality of caregiving

2. Morality: relationship to counseling, therapy, and depth psychology

The five publications that Kitwood mentioned in the Leverhulme proposal had already provided a major challenge to the medical model of dementia and set out his own "dialectical model." Also introduced was the notion of *malignant social psychology*—a term that Kitwood adopted to describe what he took to be the pathogenic nature of much dementia care provision at the time. Kitwood (1990b) argued that much of the "problem behavior" attributed to people with dementia does not arise from an internal disease process in the brain—as proposed in the medical model of dementia—but from emotional ill-being. Kitwood suggested that this ill-being is often due to the negative and inappropriate responses of care workers. The psychosocial environment surrounding people with dementia is, in Kitwood's view, often "malignant" and exacerbates rather than alleviates the symptoms of cognitive impairment. In effect, care workers often can make people with dementia worse rather than make them better. This is rarely, if ever, the result of malign intent on the part of care workers. Kitwood believed that it arises from two main sources:

1. Traditions of caregiving in dementia based on, at best, routine "behavior management" techniques and, at worst, on the mere "warehousing" of people with dementia until they die

2. Care workers' own unconscious fears about aging, disability, and death (Kitwood & Benson, 1995)

Kitwood eventually went on to identify 17 types, or manifestations, of malignant social psychology, including treachery, banishment, mockery, and objectification. A very common form of malignant social psychology is ignoring—that is, talking about people with dementia in their presence as though they are not there. Kitwood believed that malignant social psychology contributes to an erosion of personhood in those with dementia. In care environments where interactions of this nature are very frequent, clients will likely enter a downward spiral of ill-being and despair (Kitwood, 1990b). In DCM, the negative interactions that indicate a malignant social psychology are coded as Personal Detractions (PDs).

Kitwood suggested, with considerable justification, that the previously mentioned body of work opened the way for a more personalized and optimistic take on caregiving (1990b). Nonetheless, these articles contained little information about the details of good care practice or the responsibility of organizations—and of society as a whole—to ensure that professional care workers are properly supported in their work. During this stage, Kitwood was clearly preoccupied with discovering what was wrong with dementia care. Frequently, he seemed to imply that this could be discovered by detailed observation of a purely dyadic relationship between care worker and client, which he believed often acts as a conduit for malignant social psychology.

It seems likely that these preoccupations, rather than any thoroughly worked-out program for implementing person-centered care, dictated DCM's initial form, with its detailed observations of the care provided in 5-minute time frames. Although the method was subsequently adjusted to add a more positive dimension, modifications tended to be add-ons or changes in terminology rather than revisions of basic premises.

Kitwood's challenge to what he termed the "standard paradigm" of dementia and dementia care gradually evolved over a number of years, reaching its culmination in *Dementia Reconsidered: The Person Comes First* (1997). This book explores much more fully the social context of care provision and the factors that contribute to well- and ill-being in people with dementia. Had this theoretical position been fully formed before DCM was developed, the method may have been framed rather differently. For example, it is diffi- cult to imagine that by 1997 Kitwood would not develop a means of evaluat- ing QOL for those with dementia that draws in some way on "hearing the voices" of people with dementia (i.e., draws on an interpretation of the expressed concerns of participants themselves). At the outset, a major part of the rationale behind DCM was the belief that it would provide a measure of QOL from the point of view of the person with dementia. In the late 1980s, it seemed widely assumed that people with cognitive impairments could not comment on their own satisfaction with services; DCM itself made no provi- sion for this, relying instead on the observer's ability to form an empathetic judgment of what the person with dementia was experiencing. Thinking on this subject progressed rapidly, however, and by the mid-1990s, there was an upsurge in work based on "hearing the voices" of people with dementia, on psychotherapeutic approaches, on reminiscence work, and on other "talk- based" approaches (Cheston, 1998; Goldsmith, 1996). Ironically, much of this work was probably inspired at least in part by the person-centered approach to dementia care that Kitwood pioneered. Yet, the DCM method was never revised to give a direct voice to participants with dementia. Had DCM been developed a decade later, there can be little doubt that it would have done so.

In *Dementia Reconsidered*, there is still a tendency to "psychologize" social factors, including the pressures and difficulties experienced by professional care workers. Kitwood's view of social psychology was eclectic, drawing on elements from various bodies of theory—notably, the ethogenic social psy- chology proposed by Harre and Secord (1972) and others, the psychodynamic approach derived initially from the work of Freud (1932) and Jung (1977), and the humanistic psychology of Rogers (1961). These different components are not always easy to reconcile at a theoretical level, nor are they consistently applied in Kitwood's model of personhood regarding the providers and the recipients of care.

Ethogenic social psychology is concerned with ways in which humans, as "social actors," define situations, construct meanings, and communicate in- tentions. Kitwood adapted this model to great effect to demonstrate how problem behaviors in dementia can be reframed as communicative acts that express preserved aspects of the person's social identity in a changed social milieu. This approach shared much with Sabat's body of work on the preser- vation of the self in people with dementia (Sabat, 2001; Sabat & Harre, 1992). When discussing the motivations of care workers, however, Kitwood over- looked the ethogenic approach, tending to draw on literature related to moral education on the one hand and psychodynamic theory on the other. Kitwood did not view the care worker as an active "meaning-maker" but as someone who acts under the influence of unconscious psychological defenses related to repressed fears of aging, mortality, dependence, and mental incapacity (Kitwood, 1994) or the neediness of an inner child (Kitwood, 1997). Yet, later work based on interviews with care assistants (Innes, 1998b) and nurses (Packer, 2000) demonstrated that an approach based on ethogenic social psychology can reveal a wealth of information about the motivations and concerns of direct care workers.

In an article published in the *Journal of Moral Education* in 1998 (i.e., written later than *Dementia Reconsidered*), Kitwood returned to the "moral development" of professional care workers as a precondition for improving care practice. Pointing out that the majority of those employed as care providers are female, Kitwood suggested that "many people enter these professions very poorly prepared *in moral terms* for the tasks that they will face; often nursing and care assistants have had *no preparation at all*" (italics added, p. 402). This statement implies two things without evidence: 1) that there is a correlation between moral development and professional status and 2) that moral development can be taught. In pointing to the need for "moral education" for care workers, Kitwood tended to marginalize the material reality of their lives and the need for improved status, rates of pay, and working conditions.

Culture does not just relate to nationality but also to "lifeworld." The lifeworld of many direct care workers has a great deal in common almost regardless of nationality. Care workers are likely to be female, to be among the lower-paid sector of the economy, to have additional domestic responsibilities and dependents, and to have few formal qualifications. In addition, any move to bring about social change through education inevitably raises the question "Who will educate the educators?" Beyond this question, of course, are many issues related to where the responsibility for poor-quality dementia care really lies.

The body of theory that is most frequently associated with the person-centered approach is humanistic psychology, which is based on the principle that each person—no matter how unacceptable his or her behavior may seem—deserves to be accepted as a person and treated with "unconditional positive regard" (Rogers, 1961). Again, Kitwood specifically applied this approach to people with dementia, not to professional care workers and family caregivers. The theoretical or moral justification for this uneven application is unclear. Direct care workers are often at the bottom of an organizational hierarchy, so they are relatively powerless and poorly paid. If they are not treated with unconditional positive regard, then it is unrealistic to expect them to offer this to others.

To review this section, it can be said that the development of Kitwood's theory during 1985–1990 was most effective in its critique of the then nearly dominant medical model of dementia. Some aspects of this criticism were successfully translated into the basic terminology of DCM. For example, the medical model of dementia considers dementia a degenerative brain disease with symptoms that originate almost solely from neuropathology. In DCM, Kitwood introduced the concept *degeneration run* (a long period of social disengagement for a person with dementia that is uninterrupted by any care intervention). Kitwood clearly implied that degeneration results as much from external factors as from damage to neurons. Similarly, DCM classifies PDs, or episodes of malignant social psychology, as mild, moderate, severe, and very severe—the same categories that usually denote the medical model's stages of dementia. At one level, it appears that a significant part of developing and popularizing DCM was a reflexive and rhetorical turning the tables on those who normally make pronouncements about dementia and carry out assessments of those affected. If so, however, DCM misses its real target, as informed proponents of the medical model are rarely involved in direct care practice and are not affected by the DCM process.

Yet, the main concerns for using DCM in practice seem to be the microanalysis of care practice and the "re-education" of direct care workers. These DCM tenets impose on the user a particular way of seeing. Not all DCM users will be comfortable with this point of view, particularly those whose humanism extends to everyone in the care setting rather than just to people with dementia.

DEVELOPMENTS IN DEMENTIA CARE MAPPING: BASE AND SUPERSTRUCTURE

As outlined in a preceding section, the extent to which DCM was theory driven from the outset is not clear. The overall impression is that the method was developed rather quickly to satisfy the requirements of a funding body (the Leverhulme Trust). However, it is also clear that there were many subsequent opportunities to revise the method to match developing theory. The book that many practitioners still regard as the epitome of person-centered care is *Person to Person: A Guide to the Care of Those with Failing Mental Powers* (Kitwood & Bredin, 1992b). This book was published in the same year as the first DCM manual. The details of the DCM method clearly were not set in stone at this time, as evidenced by the rapid production of seven editions of the DCM manual between 1992 and 1997. Yet, the revisions seem to have been of two main types: 1) refinements in the coding techniques and data processing operations and 2) incorporation of feedback from experienced users on the mapping process.

The speed and frequency of new editions of the manual demonstrate responsiveness to the problems arising from DCM in practice. However, this response took the form of a growing number of operational rules and footnotes in successive editions rather than a revisiting of DCM's underlying premises. Later editions of the manual have a growing superstructure of rules, footnotes, and cross-references designed to deal with anomalous cases that were not anticipated at the outset. This has made DCM rather cumbersome to use and increases the potential for inaccuracy.

From about 1995 on, experienced mappers began to report significant concerns about the difficulty of achieving measurable improvements in what were then called care scores (now WIB scores) when using DCM for internal development. Reducing the overall number of PDs and negative care scores appears to have been widely accepted as an achievable target. Nevertheless, the effect of positive care interventions, even those involving Herculean efforts on the part of staff, seemed to be lost in the overall quality-of-care indices. Statistically, of course, it becomes increasingly difficult to improve any score measured on a finite scale the higher that score rises. This can be a problem when DCM is used developmentally—that is, when it is regularly repeated in the same care setting. Staff can find themselves working against an increasing "gradient" of management expectations; at the same time, the more data that are collected, the more likely is a statistical regression to the mean. Staff teams can easily become discouraged under these conditions. This was one of the concerns that led to the U.K. Study Day on DCM in 1996 and to the subsequent launch of the seventh edition of the DCM manual in May 1997. One of the most significant changes in the manual's seventh edition was the introduction of WIB values and WIB scores in place of the care values (CVs) and care scores that had been central to DCM coding in every previous edition.

At the practice level, this change was at best a compromise. It acknowledged—at least in principle—the justified feeling of many DCM users that QOL in dementia is multifactorial rather than attributable to the minute-by-minute interventions of direct care staff. Nonetheless, it did too little to make improved scores realistically achievable. The old indices remained intact, albeit with different names. Positive Event Records (PERs) were introduced as a balance to the PDs that had been a feature of DCM from the outset, but this had no effect on DCM's tendency to absorb striking examples of good care practice into overall run-of-the-mill indices of quality of care. Little emphasis was placed on these examples of affirmative practice. Although it is well established that staff are most likely to implement new approaches when they are given positive feedback and constructive suggestions (Horwath & Morrison, 1999), the section of the 97-page DCM manual allocated to PERs consists of just 2 pages.

CONCLUSION

Since the early 1990s, DCM has made a unique contribution to the evaluation of dementia care services. It has done this by putting the experience of the person with dementia in its rightful place at the forefront of attention. DCM highlighted the need for developments in care provision with the potential to maximize the well-being of this particular group of service users. It also recognized that the voices of people with dementia are likely to be unheard or discounted because of the individuals' cognitive disabilities and because of the prevailing culture of gloom and despondency that surrounded dementia care for so long. DCM challenged the view that there was "no cure, no help, no hope" for people with dementia (Kitwood & Benson, 1995). It did so primarily by accentuating the concept of experiential well-being rather than the concept of inevitable cognitive decline that is inherent in the medical model of dementia. For all of these reasons, DCM has tremendous potential for application across cultures.

In tracing the theoretical origins of DCM, three distinct strands have emerged. The first is the critique of the medical model advanced by Kitwood. This critique was instrumental in changing perceptions of both the person with dementia and the nature of dementia itself, attributing a much more significant role to the person's environment, relationships, and emotional well-being. The second is the humanistic and holistic approach to the person with dementia that is based on recognition, empathy, warmth, and acceptance of the whole person. This approach has rightly been viewed as a breakthrough in terms of its implications for dementia care practice. The third—and less frequently discussed—strand of theory relates to the moral development of care staff. This theoretical framework appears to have been uppermost in Kitwood's mind when the DCM method was developed. It has been argued in this chapter that the methodological standpoint adopted by Kitwood at this time was less firmly grounded than may have been expected in ideas related to person-centered care. On the whole, these ideas seem to have influenced slightly later work. The development of DCM appears to owe more to theories of moral education and moral development—a subject of Kitwood's (1977) own doctoral thesis.

A *methodological standpoint* can be described as a set of unspoken assumptions that inform the choice of research questions, the selection of methods, and the interpretation of findings. A number of the current limitations of

DCM can be attributed to an overemphasis of the influence that direct care staff have on overall quality of care or client well-being. Quality of care also incorporates the moral actions of management, organizations, statutory services, and government agencies. Ultimately, it is inherent in forms of social organization. It is a feature of most forms of social organization that care work is undervalued, is physically and emotionally demanding, and offers little opportunity for career progression. Working with care staff to bring about improvements in care practice should involve a commitment to recognizing and respecting their personhood and to meeting them on their territory.

REFERENCES

Audit Commission. (2000). *Forget me not: Mental health services for older people.* London: Author.

Bradford Dementia Group. (1997). *Evaluating dementia care: The DCM method* (7th ed.). Bradford, England: University of Bradford.

Cheston, R. (1998). Psychotherapeutic work with people with dementia: A review of the literature. *British Journal of Medical Psychology, 71,* 211–231.

Fothergill, A. (1989). *Heart of darkness.* Buckingham, England: Open University Press.

Freud, S. (1932). *New introductory lectures on psychoanalysis.* New York: W.W. Norton.

Goldsmith, M. (1996). *Hearing the voice of people with dementia: Opportunities and obstacles.* London: Jessica Kingsley Publishers.

Harre, R., & Secord, P.F. (1972). *The explanation of social behaviour.* Oxford, England: Blackwell Publishers.

Horwath, J., & Morrison, T. (1999). *Effective staff training in social care.* London: Routledge.

Innes, A. (1998a). Behind labels: What makes behaviour "difficult"? *Journal of Dementia Care, 6*(4), 22–25.

Innes, A. (1998b). Who cares about care assistant work? *Journal of Dementia Care, 6*(6), 33–37.

Jung, C.G. (1977). Psychological types. In G. Adler & M. Fordham (Eds.), *Collected works of C.G. Jung* (Vol. 6). Princeton, NJ: Princeton University Press.

Kitwood, T. (1977). *Values in adolescent life: Towards a critical description.* Unpublished doctoral thesis, University of Bradford, England.

Kitwood, T. (1990a). *Concern for others: A new psychology of conscience and morality.* London: Routledge.

Kitwood, T. (1990b). The dialectics of dementia with particular reference to Alzheimer's disease. *Ageing and Society, 10,* 177–196.

Kitwood, T. (1991). *The development of a method for evaluating dementia care through interaction mapping.* Unpublished extant grant application to the Leverhulme Trust, London.

Kitwood, T. (1994). Lowering our defences by playing the part. *Journal of Dementia Care, 2*(5), 12–14.

Kitwood, T. (1997). *Dementia reconsidered: The person comes first.* Buckingham, England: Open University Press.

Kitwood, T. (1998). Professional and moral development for care work: Some observations on the process. *Journal of Moral Education, 27*(3), 401–411.

Kitwood, T., & Benson, S. (1995). *The new culture of dementia care.* London: Hawker Publications.

Kitwood, T., & Bredin, K. (1992a). A new approach to the evaluation of dementia care. *Journal of Advances in Health and Nursing Care, 1*(5), 41–60.

Kitwood, T., & Bredin, K. (1992b). *Person to person: A guide to the care of those with failing mental powers.* Loughton, England: Gale Centre Publications.

McLaren, C., Mellors, C., & Radtke, D. (1991). *Faculty of social sciences: Directory of expertise.* Bradford, England: University of Bradford.

Packer, T. (2000). Attitudes towards dementia care: Education and morale in health care teams. In T. Adams & C. Clark (Eds.), *Dementia care: Partnerships in practice* (pp. 325–349). London: Ballière Tindall.

Rogers, C. (1961). *On becoming a person.* Boston: Houghton Mifflin.

Sabat, S. R. (2001). *The experience of Alzheimer's disease: Life through a tangled veil.* Oxford, England: Blackwell Publishers.

Sabat, S. R., & Harre, R. (1992). The construction and deconstruction of self in Alzheimer's disease. *Ageing and Society, 12,* 443–461.

2

THE RELIABILITY
AND VALIDITY OF
DEMENTIA CARE
MAPPING

BOB WOODS and

TRACEY LINTERN

The popularity of Dementia Care Mapping (DCM) continues to grow, fueled by positive commendations from official sources (e.g., Audit Commission, 2000). As a result, a growing number of enthusiastic practitioners attempt to use the method in their services for people with dementia. Sooner or later, many of these practitioners will face a question—probably from professionals with experience in other types of assessment instruments—along the lines of "This Dementia Care Mapping is all well and good, but is it reliable and valid?"

Similarly, as DCM is used increasingly in research and audit projects, research workers also seek reassurance that DCM possesses these hallmarks of research respectability. It is common in research papers to find reliability and validity coefficients quoted for a variety of measures, as if these features are an

We gratefully acknowledge the support of the Royal Surgical Aid Society Age-Care for the study that we carried out, which is described in this chapter.

intrinsic property of the instrument or scale. Unfortunately, this is mislead-
ing. For any measure, reliability and validity depend fundamentally on the
context in which it is used, who administers it, with whom it is being used,
and the purpose for which it is being used. Thus, the accurate answer to the
previously posed question about reliability and validity is simply but incon-
clusively, "It all depends!"

Nonetheless, this chapter aims to show the extent to which DCM *can* be
reliable and valid. It attempts to highlight some ways that practitioners can
maximize these features in their application by making clear certain factors on
which reliability and validity depend. In discussing each of these properties
in turn, their potential significance in relation to the application of DCM is
considered. It is tempting to think that such esoteric matters are the proper
concern of the researcher and the academic rather than of the practitioner. This
chapter aims to provide the practitioner with the information needed to make
an informed response to the initial question of whether DCM is reliable and
valid before returning to more important matters of person-centered care.

RELIABILITY

There are several types of reliability. In DCM, interrater reliability is often of
immediate concern. If two raters are both mapping—that is, simultaneously
observing the same people with dementia—to what extent will their maps be
consistent with each other? Would it make any difference if one rater's observations were used rather than another's? The importance of this form of reliability strongly depends on the intended use of DCM. If the intention is simply to provide feedback (via the DCM results) to the staff group to generate
ideas regarding improving the general quality of care, then precise measurement may not be critical.

Suppose that someone at a health clinic is weighed on two scales. If both
show that the person is overweight and the outcome is a discussion of ways in
which the person could exercise more and eat a healthier diet, then the fact
that the scales do not agree exactly is not important. It becomes a problem,
however, when the person returns 3 months later to monitor his or her weight
loss; it will now be difficult to determine how much change has occurred
unless the comparisons are made of weights on the same scales (and no one has
adjusted them in the meantime). If one set of scales had originally suggested
that the person was an appropriate weight for his or her height and the other
had indicated that the individual was seriously overweight, then this discrep-
ancy could have prevented the person from making needed lifestyle changes.
Similarly, interrater reliability becomes an issue for DCM 1) when it is likely

that changes over time will be of interest or 2) when the scores are being used to make comparisons with other care environments or with the DCM manual's guidelines regarding score ranges and their implications.

Retest reliability is also relevant to DCM. It reflects the extent to which maps in the same environment would be similar a few days or perhaps a week apart—that is, within a time frame when significant changes in the care environment or in the residents would not be anticipated. This aspect of reliability is again relevant for comparisons between settings or over time. If different results would be obtained if the mapping were carried out a few days later, then little importance can be attached to changes observed over a longer period or to one home's having a higher dementia care index than another. Low retest reliability can occur when interrater reliability is satisfactory and may reflect the sensitivity of the behaviors and attributes being observed to external influences. For example, the length of a piece of metal can be accurately measured, with different raters agreeing precisely on its length. On a hotter day, its length may be measured differently by the same raters because of the metal's expansion, indicating the sensitivity of the metal to ambient temperature. In dementia care, such influences may include different members of staff, a bout of acute illness among residents, or a special event in the home (e.g., party, concert, day trip).

Evidence for the Reliability of DCM

Three published substantive research studies involving DCM give some indication of interrater reliability. Brooker, Foster, Banner, Payne, and Jackson (1998) reported on a major audit project in which DCM was used in a number of professional care environments over a 3-year period. They stated that each participating observer jointly mapped with an Advanced Evaluator until a concordance coefficient (a measure of agreement, where 0 is no agreement and 1 is perfect agreement) of at least 0.8 between the mapper and the Advanced Evaluator was attained. Innes and Surr (2001) also described achieving a minimum level of concordance, before the mapping process commenced, in their report of using DCM in six residential/nursing facilities. In their study, the minimum level of concordance was 70% during the course of a 1-hour reliability test. They calculated concordance by dividing actual agreement between raters by the maximum possible agreement. Ballard and colleagues (2001) reported the use of DCM to evaluate the care environment in 10 residential/nursing facilities from the independent sector and seven from the U.K. National Health Service (NHS). They reported that all of their mappers achieved kappa scores of 0.8 and greater during a 6-hour evaluation with a senior mapper. Kappa is a commonly used index of reliability for measures of this type. It reflects the degree of agreement between raters in their choice of category for each observation period (Bowling, 1995).

None of the three studies elaborated on which of the various coding frames the reliability coefficients were calculated. This information would be of some interest. For example, it may be easier to achieve agreement on Behaviour Category Codes (BCC) than on the more subjective Well- or Ill-Being (WIB) value for each 5-minute time period observed. It would also be helpful to know whether Personal Detractions (PDs) and positive events were included. More than one of these incidences can be recorded in a 5-minute interval, so it would be difficult to specify the maximum possible agreement (Note: These elements are not included in the reliability calculations given in the seventh edition of the DCM manual [Bradford Dementia Group, 1997].) When reliability includes WIB values, percentage agreement is not ideal for calculating reliability, as it does not account for degrees of disagreement. For example, suppose that one rater records a WIB value of +3 and another rater records +1; this disagreement is less serious than if the values recorded were +3 and −1 respectively. Weighted kappa is more appropriate when the extent of disagreement is important.

A criterion of 70% agreement, as suggested by the seventh edition of the DCM manual (Bradford Dementia Group, 1997), allows the possibility of disagreements between raters in nearly one in three judgments and might be considered fairly lax. The manual acknowledges that although this level might be appropriate for developmental evaluations, higher levels are required in research studies. Breaking down reliability by individual coding frames and by behaviors within the BCC frame would enable 1) frequently occurring disagreements to be identified and 2) further operational criteria and definitions to be developed to allow a more consistent application of the measure between raters.

Although there is some evidence regarding interrater reliability, no reports in the literature regarding the retest reliability of DCM have been identified. Overall, the current evidence base for the reliability of DCM appears to be lacking, although there are some encouraging indications.

Maximizing the Reliability of Dementia Care Mapping

A number of steps may be taken to enhance the reliability of any observational method. First, each behavior to be recorded should be clearly defined, with notations of how it is distinct from other similar behaviors, to avoid ambiguity. Subjective judgments should be reduced to a minimum. The extensive development work on and multiple revisions of the DCM manual have gone a long way to ensure such clarity. By their very nature, WIB ratings involve a subjective element, and this evaluative element is a cardinal feature of DCM (Brooker, 1995); however, through clear definitions and numerous examples, agreement between raters in this area also should be possible.

Second, mappers must be trained so that they understand the DCM procedure and behavior definitions and have the opportunity to work through examples with experienced mappers. A 3-day training course, including an introduction to person-centered care, remains mandatory for dementia care mappers. This requirement represents good practice in the field. As suggested previously, a particular aim of DCM training should be to ensure one's understanding of and agreement with expert raters regarding WIB values.

Third, extensive practice is essential to developing proficiency in any observational method. Many of those who successfully complete training in DCM do not conduct sufficient maps to become thoroughly familiar with DCM's method and definitions in actual practice. Generally speaking, reliability can be enhanced by using more experienced raters, especially when these raters undertake regular reliability checks, as encouraged by the DCM manual. This component is important, as it is possible for mappers to gradually develop idiosyncratic interpretations of definitions and criteria if they do not regularly check their ratings with those of other observers.

Fourth, reliability of any observational method is generally greater when the number of potential categories to be recorded is low. A greater number of behavioral categories to remember makes it more difficult to secure agreement between raters. DCM has a relatively high number of categories, especially when the 17 types of PDs are also considered. Efforts have been made to ease the memorization of the categories and their attendant codes. Yet, there are also some decision rules to remember (e.g., daytime sleeping attracts a more negative WIB value as time progresses, a precedence of certain categories exists if several occur in a time interval), so it is clear that DCM requires more memorization than most other observational methods in dementia care. Nonetheless, the time frame (5 minutes) during which observations are made is relatively generous and usually allows time to consider the appropriate category.

Fifth, reliability is also generally greater when there is less activity in the area being observed. This factor influences how many residents may be observed. Innes and Surr (2001) reported mapping 5–10 residents simultaneously. When more residents come and go from the observation area or a greater number of interactions occur, there will inevitably be a decrease in the number of residents who can be satisfactorily observed. Of course, if the 10 residents being observed are all dozing in a lounge, then interrater reliability will be high!

Sixth, in observational studies, disagreements between raters often occur because one has a better view of a particular incident than another. Finding a good location from which to observe unobtrusively is essential for reliable ratings. Nevertheless, this is not an easy task, especially in care environments that are more homey in scale and design.

Seventh, observation is hard work, and reliability of recording may suffer when the rater becomes tired or feels uneasy regarding what is being observed. Brooker suggested, "It can be an extremely uncomfortable experience to carry out an observational study in an environment where care is poor" (1995, p. 154). Regular breaks during the mapping and opportunities to debrief with another mapper (to enable mutual support) are essential for maintaining the quality of mapping.

VALIDITY

In essence, the validity of any measure reflects the extent to which it does indeed measure what it sets out to measure. A number of types of validity are distinguished (e.g., see Bowling, 1997). *Content validity* determines whether the measure adequately covers the totality of the area. One aspect of content validity is *face validity*, the extent to which the measure transparently evaluates the aspects it is intended to measure. Face validity ascertains whether the measure's relevance and appropriateness are readily recognized by users of the method. *Criterion validity* determines how the measure relates to the "gold standard"—that is, the best measure that is currently available. *Concurrent validity* involves using the measure alongside existing measures and evaluating their degree of correlation. *Predictive validity* evaluates how well the measure predicts future differences (e.g., Does the DCM WIB index predict which residents a visiting clinician will diagnose as being depressed?). *Construct validity* tests theoretical associations to build a picture of the measure's validity and its underlying theory. For example, it might be predicted that facilities with lower dementia care indices have higher rates of psychotropic medication use or that less mobile residents have lower WIB scores. These examples demonstrate *convergent validity*, when theoretically related variables are expected to show correlations with each other.

Consideration of DCM's validity is complicated because the measure appears to evaluate several attributes:

1. Relative amount of time spent in various activities

2. Average WIB value for each person with dementia

3. Average across the care environment of WIB values for each person with dementia

4. Distribution of WIB scores across all people with dementia observed, indicating which proportion of observations falls into each of the six WIB categories

5. The unit-wide dementia care index, which reflects a combination of Attribute 3 and the diversity of positive activities from the BCC list in which residents engaged (a weighted dementia care index, adjusted to account for the ratio of staff to residents, may also be calculated, although this is rarely practiced)

The foci of certain studies on DCM demonstrate how the method can measure these various attributes. For example, Ballard and colleagues (2001) reported on Attributes 3 and 5; Brooker and colleagues (1998) reported on Attributes 3 and 4 and used the BCC data for Attribute 1; and Innes and Surr (2001) reported on Attributes 2, 3, and 4 together, with some aspects of Attribute 1. In addition, the latter two studies reported figures for PDs also. Within this range of measures and indices, a fundamental distinction can be drawn between the use of DCM to describe 1) the individual with dementia, his or her range of activities, and his or her degree of well- or ill-being and 2) the quality of a care environment. Thus, the distinction is between quality of life (QOL) and quality of care. In the seventh edition of DCM manual, Kitwood pointed out that although a broad correspondence may be anticipated between these aspects, they will diverge in a number of scenarios. For example, people with mild dementia sometimes overcome deficient care and maintain a high level of well-being by drawing on their own resources; conversely, physical health problems or long-standing psychological disorders may lead to relative ill-being despite good-quality care. In considering the validity of DCM, it is often helpful to distinguish validity at the level of the individual resident from validity at a unit level.

Findings from Research Studies on the Validity of Dementia Care Mapping

Face and content validity are evident from DCM's development, which has included feedback from users, and from the widespread acceptance of DCM as the gold standard. In their 3-year audit project, Brooker and colleagues (1998) administered a Staff Acceptability Questionnaire, and 260 questionnaires were completed over the three 1-year cycles. By the third cycle, 100% of respondents thought that mapping results would be useful in improving care (compared with 88% initially); only 10% reported anxiety about the evaluation (compared with 22% initially).

Concurrent validity is reflected at a unit level by the relationship of DCM unit measures with other environmental quality measures. However, although such measures were used in at least two studies (Brooker et al., 1998; Lintern, Woods, & Phair, 2000a, 2000b), they were used to compare individual WIB scores with the comparison measure rather than to make an aggregate comparison over a number of units. For example, Brooker and colleagues evaluated levels of engagement using a time-sample methodology similar to that used by Jenkins, Felce, Lunt, and Powell (1977) to evaluate the quality of care environments. In this methodology, a decision is made whether the person is engaged or disengaged (actively interacting with the environment or not) during a 20-second period every 5 minutes. Brooker and colleagues recorded levels of engagement for 10 people with dementia across a 6-hour period. Recordings were contemporaneous with the usual DCM method, which resulted in an individual WIB value that could be correlated with the percentage of observations in which the person was engaged. For these 10 individuals, the WIB values and percentage engagement were highly correlated (correlation coefficient $r = 0.80$; significance level $p = 0.01$).

In our own longitudinal study of a training and development program in a nursing facility (Lintern, Woods, & Phair, 2000a, 2000b), we used another observational procedure—the extended version of the Quality of Interactions Schedule (QUIS; Dean, Proudfoot, & Lindesay, 1993). Like engagement scores, this procedure has been used to compare different care environments regarding the percentage of interactions recorded between staff and residents, which are rated as being of positive quality. We extended the range of positive interactions that could be recorded so that, for example, an extended conversation would be scored higher than a brief greeting; then, we recorded interactions for each resident separately. This meant that each resident's experience of interactions with staff was recorded and could be compared with his or her WIB value from DCM. Forty-seven residents were observed using both DCM and the extended QUIS (see Table 2.1). The observations were not simultaneous; some were made a few weeks apart. Positive correlations were found between residents' WIB values and staff's having conversations with them, as well as with staff's talking to the resident (i.e., more than a few words) during personal care. These findings only emerged on the extended QUIS categories; the original QUIS criteria (developed in a hospital context) required only a few words and are too insensitive for residential/nursing facilities.

We also administered the Life Experiences Checklist (LEC; Ager, 1990). LEC is a 50-item checklist designed to measure important but possibly infrequent aspects of life, indicating the extent to which each resident is able to participate in the kind of activities that most people value (e.g., taking trips, having contact with family, having a pleasant home). The LEC includes five subscales: 1) Home, 2) Leisure, 3) Relationships, 4) Freedom, and 5) Opportunities; a total score may also be calculated. Staff members who knew the resident well completed this checklist from the person's perspective. Two of the

Table 2.1. Correlations of Dementia Care Mapping (DCM) Well- and Ill-Being values with the extended Quality of Interactions Schedule (QUIS; Dean, Proudfoot, & Lindesay, 1993)

Extended QUIS	Correlation with DCM
Positive social–conversation (>2 minutes)	0.48[a]
Positive social–verbal (>7 words)	0.19
Positive social–brief (<7 words)	0.14
Positive care–conversation	0.34[b]
Positive care–verbal	0.32[b]
Positive care–brief	0.22
Neutral	–0.15
Negative protective	–0.10
Negative restrictive	0.10

$N = 47$
[a] significant at $p = 0.001$; [b] significant at $p = 0.05$

subscales showed a significant correlation with individual WIB values for 42 residents for whom both measures were available (see the top portion of Table 2.2). Leisure and Opportunities were also the subscales with the lowest average scores. It may be that the lack of correlation with some other subscales (especially Home) reflects the uniformity of living environment for most residents. The correlations between some LEC scores and WIB values are especially important in view of the different time frames they evaluate. One criticism of DCM is that it may miss significant events in the person's life that occur outside the 2 days of mapping. The once-weekly trip to a pub with a relative or participation in an annual holiday's festivities, for example, would contribute to LEC scores but not to DCM, so the degree of overlap between the two measures is useful evidence for the validity of DCM.

In relation to construct validity, a number of relationships between variables may be of interest in establishing convergent validity. Brooker and colleagues (1998) examined the association of Clifton Assessment Procedure for the Elderly (CAPE) Dependency scores and individual WIB scores. The survey version of the CAPE (Pattie & Gilleard, 1979) assesses the person's level of dependency and was completed by staff prior to each cycle of mapping. In the first two cycles, there was a significant correlation between WIB and CAPE scores (–0.7 and –0.63), such that higher levels of dependency were associated with lower WIB values. This association reduced greatly at the third DCM cycle ($r = -0.25$), suggesting that by this stage, ways of increasing well-being were emphasized for patients who were highly dependent.

In our study, we evaluated functional abilities using the Adaptive Behaviour Rating Scale (ABRS; Ward, Murphy, & Procter, 1991; Woods & Britton,

Table 2.2.　Correlations of Dementia Care Mapping Well- and Ill-Being (WIB) values with the Life Experiences Checklist (LEC; Ager, 1990), the Depressive Signs Scale (Katona & Aldridge, 1985), and the Adaptive Behaviour Rating Scale (ABRS; Woods & Britton, 1985)

LEC, Depressive Signs Scale, and ABRS values	Correlation with WIB values	Sample size
LEC–Home	0.09	42
LEC–Leisure	0.35[a]	42
LEC–Relationships	0.16	42
LEC–Freedom	0.14	42
LEC–Opportunities	0.32[a]	42
LEC–TOTAL	0.29	42
Depressive Signs Scale	−0.36[a]	47
ABRS–Dressing	0.28	47
ABRS–Personal Hygiene	0.29[a]	47
ABRS–Eating	0.28	47
ABRS–Mobility	0.29[a]	47
ABRS–Communication	0.03	47
ABRS–Toilet requirements	0.20	47
ABRS–Recognition of others	0.47[c]	45
ABRS–Orientation	0.42[b]	46
ABRS–Activity Disturbance	0.01	47
ABRS–Aggressivity	−0.31[a]	47

[a]significant at $p = 0.05$; [b]significant at $p = 0.01$; [c]significant at $p = 0.001$

1985), which enabled us to evaluate the association of individual WIB values with the profile of the person's functional capacity. The ABRS was completed by staff who knew the resident well. Generally, higher WIB scores were associated with lower levels of impairment (see the lower portion Table 2.2). This finding was significant in relation to personal hygiene and mobility; cognitive aspects, such as orientation and recognition of others, showed the highest degree of association. It is interesting to note that communication difficulties were not related to WIB values. Residents who showed higher levels of physical and verbal aggression had lower WIB values, reflecting the impact of disturbance and distress on well-being. The Depressive Signs Scale (Katona & Aldridge, 1985) was also administered. This is a validated measure of depression that staff complete, as it focuses on the observable signs of depression rather than on self-report. Residents who had higher levels of depression had significantly lower WIB values (see Table 2.2).

Future Research Considerations for the Validity of Dementia Care Mapping

The previous subsection reviewed evidence indicating that individual WIB values are associated with engagement and quality of interaction recordings from other observational methods, as well as that there are a number of significant correlations with measures of depression, current life experiences, and functional level. More evidence is needed in all of these areas, however, especially in relation to the association with levels of dependency. Raising WIB values of people with low dependency to an extent that reduces the association between WIB values and dependency has important implications for raising quality of care for those with the highest dependency levels. There has been considerable development work on QOL measures for people with dementia that can be completed with the person (e.g., the Quality of Life in Alzheimer's Disease [QOL-AD]; Logsdon, Gibbons, McCurry, & Teri, 1999). Comparisons of scores on these measures with WIB values would be of great interest.

Some evidence is emerging that supports the validity of the individual WIB values, but little appears to be known regarding overall ratings of environmental quality using DCM. For example, Ballard and colleagues (2001) reported dementia care indices for 17 care environments. They concluded that care standards are low because all were rated as needing "radical changes" or "much improvement" based on the score ranges given in the seventh edition of the DCM manual. However, it is not clear how these score ranges and descriptors were derived. No norms as such are provided in the manual, although presumably these score ranges were based on extensive experience of the method. In Ballard's study, the NHS facilities appeared to offer the worst quality of care (all required "radical changes"), but the lower ratings may reflect the fact that the residents in these care settings were more impaired (cognitively and behaviorally) than those in other settings. Studies are needed that compare a large number of care settings of variable quality on DCM indices and other environmental measures, such as the Multiphasic Environmental Assessment Procedure scales developed by Moos and Lemke (1984) or those developed by Bowie, Mountain, and Clayden (1992).

More consideration could also be given to whether DCM is an effective vehicle for change—for improving the quality of care. Does it highlight areas of change that have a real impact on the experiences and QOL of people with dementia? Is it a valid tool for this purpose? Several studies have suggested that feedback on DCM, leading to an action plan that is developed and implemented by staff, leads to observable changes. For the most part, however, these changes have been evaluated by a further round of DCM (e.g., Barnett, 2000;

Brooker et al., 1998; Lintern, Woods, & Phair, 2000a, 2000b) and provide little evidence from other sources to support the changes. Our study did show that staff attitudes and care skills increased, but much of this change appeared to follow staff training rather than DCM feedback and action planning.

Furthermore, additional research is needed regarding the interaction of certain aspects of DCM and its validity. First, mapping only takes place in public areas of care units for sound ethical reasons. Does this factor limit the validity of the method? Is care that is provided in private of a different quality than that on view in public areas? If residents increasingly choose to spend time in their own rooms, will it become increasingly difficult to map validly? Of course, these are issues for any observational method.

In addition, it would be helpful to have more information regarding the extent of mapping that is required to give a valid picture for an individual or for an environment as a whole. Because 2 days of observations are generally required, cost is often cited as a reason for not using DCM. Is a day enough time? An hour? Or, are 2 days actually insufficient for obtaining a valid assessment of the care environment or the individual's well-being? The latter may especially show a great deal of day-to-day fluctuation, and as mentioned previously, DCM is not designed to evaluate infrequent but important positive or negative events in the person's life, which may have considerable bearing on QOL.

Finally, as with all observational methods, people with dementia and staff may behave differently when an observer is present. As Brooker commented, all that the observer may be doing is "looking at them, looking at me" (1995, p. 145); by the observer's very presence, the situation ceases to be normal or typical. This factor can be addressed by continuing to map over an extended period and comparing results from early and late in the process. It is predicted that reactivity effects would lessen over time. Nonetheless, despite many mappers' belief that no one put on an act for them, it is difficult to be certain of the extent of this effect without further validation through methods that use nonobservational methodologies.

CONCLUSION

The evidence on the reliability and validity of DCM has yet to do justice to the richness of the approach. Although some encouraging evidence is already available, significant gaps in knowledge exist. Care must be taken to inform users that findings for one use of DCM do not necessarily generalize to other applications.

REFERENCES

Ager, A. (1990). *Life Experiences Checklist*. Windsor, England: NFER-Nelson.

Audit Commission. (2000). *Forget me not: Mental health services for older people*. London: Author.

Ballard, C., Fossey, J., Chithramohan, R., Howard, R., Burns, A., Thompson, P., Tadros, G., & Fairbairn, A. (2001). Quality of care in private sector and NHS facilities for people with dementia: cross-sectional survey. *British Medical Journal, 323,* 426–427.

Barnett, E. (2000). *Including the person with dementia in designing and delivering care: 'I need to be me!'* London: Jessica Kingsley Publishers.

Bowie, P., Mountain, G., & Clayden, D. (1992). Assessing the environmental quality of long-stay wards for the confused elderly. *International Journal of Geriatric Psychiatry, 7,* 95–104.

Bowling, A. (1995). *Measuring disease*. Buckingham, England: Open University Press.

Bowling, A. (1997). *Measuring health* (2nd ed.). Buckingham, England: Open University Press.

Bradford Dementia Group. (1997). *Evaluating dementia care: The DCM method* (7th ed.). Bradford, England: University of Bradford.

Brooker, D. (1995). Looking at them, looking at me: A review of observational studies into the quality of institutional care for elderly people with dementia. *Journal of Mental Health, 4,* 145–156.

Brooker, D., Foster, N., Banner, A., Payne, M., & Jackson, L. (1998). The efficacy of dementia care mapping as an audit tool: Report of a 3-year British NHS evaluation. *Aging & Mental Health, 2,* 60–70.

Dean, R., Proudfoot, R., & Lindesay, J. (1993). The Quality of Interactions Schedule (QUIS): Development, reliability, and use in the evaluation of two domus units. *International Journal of Geriatric Psychiatry, 8,* 819–826.

Innes, A., & Surr, C. (2001). Measuring the well-being of people with dementia living in formal care settings: the use of dementia care mapping. *Aging & Mental Health, 5,* 258–268.

Jenkins, J., Felce, D., Lunt, B., & Powell, E. (1977). Increasing activity of residents in old people's homes by providing recreational materials. *Behaviour Research and Therapy, 15,* 429–434.

Katona, C.L.E., & Aldridge, C.R. (1985). The dexamethasone suppression test and depressive signs in dementia. *Journal of Affective Disorders, 8,* 83–89.

Lintern, T., Woods, B., & Phair, L. (2000a). Before and after training: A case study of intervention. *Journal of Dementia Care, 8*(1), 15–17.

Lintern, T., Woods, B., & Phair, L. (2000b). Training is not enough to change care practice. *Journal of Dementia Care, 8*(2), 15–17.

Logsdon, R., Gibbons, L.E., McCurry, S.M., & Teri, L. (1999). Quality of life in Alzheimer's disease: Patient and caregiver reports. *Journal of Mental Health and Aging, 5*(1), 21-32.

Moos, R.H., & Lemke, S. (1984). *Multiphasic Environmental Assessment Procedure.* Stanford, CA: Stanford University Press.

Pattie, A., & Gilleard, C.J. (1979). *Manual of the Clifton Assessment Procedures for the Elderly.* London: Hodder & Stoughton.

Ward, T., Murphy, E., & Procter, A. (1991). Functional assessment in severely demented patients. *Age and Ageing, 20,* 212–216.

Woods, R.T., & Britton, P.G. (1985). *Clinical psychology with the elderly.* London: Croom Helm.

3

USING DEMENTIA CARE MAPPING IN HEALTH AND SOCIAL CARE SETTINGS

LISA HELLER

*A vision without
a task is a dream.
A task without
a vision is drudgery.
But a vision with
a task can change
the world.*
*—Attributed to
Black Elk (1863–1950),
Chief of the Oglala Sioux*

With reference to Dementia Care Mapping (DCM), the word *culture* can simply be defined as "the way we do things." Yet, examining portions of some dictionary definitions of the term reveals considerable diversity. *The Little Oxford Dictionary* (Waite, 1998) defines *culture* as "intellectual and artistic achievement or expression," while the *New Oxford Dictionary of English* (Pearsall, 2001) definition reads, "trained and refined state of the understanding and manners and tastes, phase of this prevalent at a time or place. Instilling of it by training." The *Merriam-Webster's Collegiate Dictionary* (1997) says that *culture* is "the integrated pattern of knowledge, belief and behavior that depends on man's capacity for learning and transmitting knowledge to succeeding generations." Finally, the *Cassell's English Dictionary* (1979) definition is "the act of tilling."

From these definitions, a wider picture of *culture* emerges. It is an "integrated pattern"—which implies learning, discipline, and training—as well as "tilling." Using DCM to bring about behavior change requires understanding of 1) the desired culture (i.e., the "new culture" of dementia care; Kitwood & Benson, 1995) and 2) the prevalent culture in each setting. Sometimes, it may be wise not to conduct DCM because of culture issues:

> *The staff team at Maple was negotiating with the DCM workers about whether to have a second map. The team felt that it was not appropriate to be mapped again because Maple cared for people who were too frail and the mappers {were} not familiar with the clients. Some staff members disliked mapping so much the first time that they said they would take sick days if a second map were to take place.*

How could the DCM workers make it acceptable to proceed with the evaluation? Understanding the basis of the staff's anxieties and their pattern of knowledge, belief, and behavior—that is, the culture of that care environment—was required. Therefore, the following steps were taken:

- Withdrawal of the planned mapping sessions was necessary for negotiation to take place under less pressure.

- The DCM team met with the care staff and discovered that their overriding expressed need was further training. None of the care staff had specific training in dementia care or in person-centered care. They felt that they were being picked on because they were not specialists. The culture in Maple had become defensive; staff were demoralized and lacked the ability or capacity to change without external help, which they resented and feared.

> *Another staff team in Rose Lea, an assessment center, was negotiating whether to have a second map. "I think we should go ahead," said a staff member. "It teaches us how it feels to be watched, which is what our clients experience."*

In this unit, sufficient numbers on the staff team were convinced of the value of DCM because they had been thoroughly prepared. Four team members, including the unit manager, were trained mappers, and the unit staff had undergone several short practice maps. The staff had also read several articles about person-centered care and DCM. The culture in the second unit was more open than the first one. The staff were used to educational and training input and felt the need for further help. A critical mass of staff was already sympathetic to the ethos of DCM and person-centered ideology.

STAFF AND CARE CULTURE CONSIDERATIONS

DCM is not value free (Bradford Dementia Group, 1997). It does not simply give a bland reflection of what is happening in a care setting. It is designed to embody certain values—those of a person-centered approach to care and care staff, both in its delivery and in the purpose for which it is used. It enables a powerful and practical understanding of what is going on within a unit for the purpose of improvement. For the change process to be effective—and for DCM not to simply put pressure on unit staff—all those involved in direct care as well as those who manage, commission care, and set standards should be engaged in the DCM process. Doctors and senior nurses have a powerful influence on the culture of the setting and, thus, should be involved. As Marshall noted, existing care training may not be sufficient: "Many registration and inspection officers and . . . managers were . . . trained well before the more optimistic models of dementia care were developed, and many remain ignorant of them" (2001, p. 410).

Considering the Culture of Care in the Setting to Be Evaluated

When a DCM evaluation is proposed for a particular environment, the mappers must be sensitive to the current culture of care. The manager of a hospital ward had worked hard to introduce person-centered care to the ward. In considering a DCM evaluation, she said,

> *Using the phrase, "New culture of dementia care," implies that our present culture is wrong. I want to convey to my team of staff that a lot of what they do is good, not that they have got to throw everything out of the window.*

This manager understood that person-centered care necessitates valuing staff and the skills that they bring to their work. She believed that DCM needed to be conducted in a way that was sensitive to such appreciation. In this situation, DCM workers did not talk about introducing a new culture but supported the culture that was already being nurtured and "tilled."

Packer suggested that there are

> Places in existence which "talk the person-centered talk" but do not "walk the person-centered walk" . . . The concerns of those care workers who are expected to "make do" with what they have on a day-to-day basis should be taken very seriously indeed. Unless they are, person-centered care is in danger of "failure to thrive" and will languish in a sea of worker burnout and apathy. (2000, pp. 19–20)

DCM can highlight the need for certain changes, and implementing these changes necessitates far-reaching developments in the culture of care that require the support of personnel throughout the organization.

INFLUENCES ON A CARE ENVIRONMENT'S CULTURE

The culture of each setting is determined by a number of factors, which are detailed next.

Society

Caregiving institutions, large and small, are subject to the cultural influence of wider society. Attitudes toward aging and toward dementia influence care provision (Kitwood, 1997). There is a tendency to view older people as less valuable and less able to contribute within the family and workplace. Ageism is endemic in many societies, where older people are seen as incompetent and burdensome. Discrimination works against them at both a personal and a structural level. Kitwood described the ways in which many cultures have a tendency to depersonalize those who have some form of disability. The use of the word "senile" dismisses even those who have dementia but who are not old. Too few resources have been made available to provide proper care for people with dementia, and specialist training for the skilled work involved in caring for people with dementia is not developed.

Institution's Ethos

Individual care units are usually part of larger organizations and tend to take their ethos from the parent institution. The terms and conditions for workers—as well as the standard practice for the treatment of clients, relatives, and visitors—are as influential as establishing regulations and setting standards.

The Unit Itself

Each unit, even if it is part of a larger institution (e.g., a ward within a hospital, a day center within an assessment unit), can usually determine its own culture in subtle yet important ways, such as surface décor (e.g., photographs, mirrors, flowers, labeling and color coding of areas and rooms, floor coverings). Routines and the use of resources are often determined by units, too. For example, music may be played; dance and movement may be encouraged. In addition, a unit may provide objects to look at, touch, soothe, or stimulate. Finally, units determine to some degree how visitors are treated. Are they welcomed or regarded as problematic?

Total Environment of the Care Setting

The architecture of the care setting has significant effects on the people receiving care as well as on care staff (Fleming, 1993). The total environment has enormous significance for the organization and delivery of care. On the one hand, a local day center that is staffed by volunteers is more likely to reflect the culture of the people receiving care than a large hospital ward. Volunteers and local workers bring their history to their work. Dialect, accent, and the meaning of words may be significant on a local scale. For example, in certain areas of England, "love" is a commonly accepted form of addressing individuals. Such terms can comfort in local surroundings but may give rise to misunderstanding in other places.

On the other hand, a hospital ward imposes its own history. It may have originally been an asylum and may possess some of the features of the old "Nightingale" wards: long rooms—with perhaps as many as 20 beds, separated by only a chair, a locker, and a curtain—and no private space. Sometimes, management of a locally built hospital nurtures opportunities provided by local understanding and invites involvement from the community. Other times, it simply replaces the old gray institution with a new pink one.

Local-Level Decisions

The following vignette demonstrates the effect of decisions made at the local level:

> As the end of the financial year approached, two units were informed that they had leftover funds in their budgets. The hospital ward ordered a weighing scale and three machines to measure blood pressure. The social care home ordered new curtains for the lounge and matching cushion covers. When it was suggested that both units could buy something for the people receiving care, the hospital ward ordered some new skirts and trousers and the social care home ordered some plants for the patio.

The plants became a focus for planting, tending, and watching. With a little prompting, that unit had been able to use its money in a creative way, which held potential for continued development.

Budget

In both health and social care settings, there are guidelines and restrictions on the use of the budget. Yet, the way that the budget is spent often reflects the unit's culture. One hospital ward decided to employ two of its support workers on a daytime shift to cover the busiest periods for that ward. A residential care home employed part-time staff who wished to work nights only. The way that even limited resources are deployed can have far-reaching effects on the culture of care.

Management

The aspirations and attitude of the manager are crucial in determining how DCM works in a unit. Outcomes from any DCM initiatives depend on the level of management's support for staff to enable engagement with feedback and the mobilization of available resources:

Following a full DCM evaluation in a social care home, some care work-ers were angry that the map indicated that one person in the unit seemed to have suffered more ill-being than other people. The care workers argued that this resident had been ill, had fallen, had slept poorly, and so forth. What did the mappers expect? Couldn't an exception be made? It appeared that the map confirmed what had been in the staff's minds. The manager pointed out agreement between what the care workers were saying and what the mapping showed. She resolved to call the doctor that day for the resi-dent to receive a proper medical checkup and to try to sort out the findings.

The manager recognized the truth of the findings. She also validated the sense of failure expressed by her staff team. She understood that the agreement between the findings and the staff's perceptions needed to be noted and that the support for both her team and for DCM required not argument but action.

Staff Team

With leadership and facilitation by the manager, the unit team can bring about considerable elements of creative change:

A health care unit's DCM evaluation determined that mealtimes were uncomfortable and difficult for everyone. In response, the unit introduced "therapeutic meals." These were specially designed mealtimes, with dedicated staff chosen for each occasion. For a carefully selected group of residents, the meal was taken in a separate dining area. The menu was chosen with the needs of the particular residents in mind—for example, finger foods, spe-cially preferred cakes, and so forth. A range of music and table decorations were made available, and no interruptions were to take place. The care workers were responsible for enabling the residents to eat as independently as possible, and they would encourage and take part in social interaction. Staff would eat their meal alongside the residents. Therapeutic mealtimes were designed to address a range of issues raised by the DCM evaluation. Staff who were normally busy—who tended to be "task orientated" and were eas-ily distracted at mealtimes—were encouraged to help and support residents. Both staff and residents would enjoy some time together, away from the bus-tle and confusion of the usual dining room, when the barriers of "us and them" would be lessened and they could engage in genuine social contact.

In this unit, the staff considered their own roles and had recognized the influ-ence of their routines and actions on those whom they served.

Individual Staff Members

Speaking about the therapeutic meals in her unit, a care worker commented, "The problem is that only the more able residents are invited to the meals, but everyone should have a chance to go. If certain residents need a bit more help, I would be happy to go in with them." Individuals can bring about some of these local, cultural changes. Given support, this worker had the potential to influence the direction that these changes would take and also influence her co-workers.

Expectations

The expectations of the care workers and clients help form the unit's style and contribute to its culture:

> A staff team in a social care unit was preparing for its first DCM evaluation. An activity was planned for the first afternoon of mapping. On the appointed day, only three residents appeared in the day room, so the activity was cancelled. The mappers were told that the residents were too tired to participate.

This example illustrates low staff and resident expectations. It was not considered a priority to develop a routine that balanced the need for rest and quiet with the need for stimulating activity.

This point is further illustrated by another example from a hospital assessment unit:

> On the day of the initial practice map, Mrs. A. gave one of her care workers a shoulder massage. During the feedback portion of DCM, the care worker said that she felt guilty about the incident. However, the mapper suggested that this staff member demonstrated a willingness to validate Mrs. A.'s desire to give something back to her care workers.

In this vignette, the mapper explained to the care worker and her colleagues that this situation made possible a giving opportunity. That is, the care worker enabled and accepted the gift that Mrs. A. was clearly glad to offer. This example illustrates an aspect of what Kitwood (1997) described as *positive person work*.

Age

Bell and McGregor (1994) described the influence of the residents on the culture within their own unit and how they were able to become part of the "group." The ages of all people in the care environment contribute to the predominant culture. Care workers and residents who are from an older generation can share memories and perhaps even sing familiar songs. Young care workers may bring joy through a unique style of dress and playfulness. Younger people with dementia may also affect the dynamic and culture of the setting; however, there may be little to interest or stimulate them in a culture that is alien to them—one that is literally from a different age.

Power Relations

Power relationships exist in all care environments for people with dementia. The unit team's hierarchy may be very strict, or it may be somewhat democratic. Pay structures, qualifications, and grades are significant factors in the way that staff see themselves within the setting. In addition, the people with dementia and their family care workers are often regarded as the recipients of a service and, thus, are given fewer opportunities for decision making, influence, and control.

Blame Culture or Inclusive Culture

A unit that has frequently received criticism and blame in previous external inspections will be influenced by this past history. As the manager of one care home remarked, "We are working in a blame culture. We've got to help the staff to see what is good about what they do instead of them always expecting to be told what they're doing wrong."

To prevent DCM from being viewed as yet another way of blaming staff, it is vital to enable care workers to reflect on past observations and to encourage their sense of empowerment. Fostering an inclusive culture is important if a care unit is to move away from a "blame culture" (Heller, 2001). An inclusive culture accepts diversity. It accepts the way that people work, with their skills and strengths as well as their weaknesses and failings. People can survive being blamed and bullied, but they will work better if they are valued and their creativity is encouraged to flourish:

> One hospital ward had received three DCM evaluations. The residents had severe disabilities and complex needs, and they engaged in frequent outbursts of frustration and anger. During one winter and early spring, local volunteers helped the ward staff create a new sensory garden. The staff were found to have a variety of useful skills for this project. Their friends and relatives also made valuable contributions. The finished garden contained benches; water features; walkways; raised beds; and a variety of plants to offer many colors, textures, and scents.

This garden was the brainchild of the ward's new manager, who developed the idea after she and four staff members trained in DCM:

> A subsequent map of the ward showed that the third most commonly observed behavior was sensory activity. When difficult incidents caused the people with dementia to become frustrated and angry, care workers

would walk with the person in the garden. Some residents were not able to walk in the garden, so edible herbs were brought inside for them to touch and smell.

The ward staff clearly felt ownership of the garden. Pride in the garden and their part in its creation launched new elements in the routine care of people in the ward and opened up new forms of creativity in responding to needs. The garden help received from local volunteers also made the care workers aware of the wider community's interest in and commitment to their work.

Summary

It is important for mappers to be able to pick up clues about the setting, which may influence how DCM is received. Individuals, groups, and dynamics within the staff team and the environment all play important parts in forming the culture of the unit.

TYPE OF CARE ENVIRONMENT AND SELF-PERCEPTION OF CARE WORKER ROLES

Social care, residential care, or day care staff may accept that helping people to eat and go to the bathroom are important aspects of their jobs. Engaging people in discussions about television shows and playing a game of soccer with active residents may also be seen as part of daily living. However, it may be harder for staff to accept the use of activities for therapy, engagement, or contact. Helping hospital ward residents with self-care activities sometimes appears to be the most important care element. Therefore, occupational diversity and engagement are extras that can be done only if and when staff numbers and time permit. As Marshall noted,

> It is all too easy to blame the dementia for the extent to which patients spend their time sleeping or sitting apathetically around the walls of the communal areas. In a sense, dementia itself lets staff at all levels, and those responsible for quality of care, off the hook. (2001, p. 411)

As a result, residents with profound disabilities are often left slumped in their chairs, which line the wall of the lounge or the ward.

Based on the impression that DCM will impose certain changes on a unit's culture, staff may either embrace or reject DCM as a whole. One staff member of an extended care hospital ward made a comment that co-workers echoed: "We are a nursing unit. DCM can help us with some things but, really, our work is to nurse these people and we can't expect any more of our staff or our clients."

Staff in a unit for people with challenging behavior tend to view all behavior as challenging. They may see their role as "dealing with" or "managing" behavior. They may contest that using DCM is unrealistic in their unit and reject any idea of improving the residents' well-being. It is almost as if the people with dementia and challenging behavior have forfeited the right to well-being. They must be cared for and kept safe, but engagement, contact, and therapy are luxuries. Keys, baffle locks, and uniforms are prominent in these settings. The unique culture of the setting, with all of its internal and external influences, is a clearer determinant of how DCM is viewed and used by staff than its label as a "health" or "social care" setting.

THE CULTURE OF DEMENTIA CARE MAPPING

> *During preparation for a DCM evaluation in a hospital assessment ward, the staff discussion centered around Personal Detractions, particularly the use of endearments and the concept of infantilization. The staff team wanted to know the role of local culture and colloquialisms. Would they get in trouble for using local words?*

This discussion raised an important issue. Does DCM seek to impose a set of values on others, which may destroy spontaneity and, possibly, the forming of worthwhile relationships? On the one hand, if a resident used to call patrons of his paper shop "dear," then having care workers call him "dear" may be comforting. On the other hand, a resident who was always called "Ms. _____" may find "dear" forward and offensive.

How Dementia Care Mapping Is Conducted

The observation component of mapping may help some care workers become more sensitive to residents, who must feel that they are being observed almost all of the time. Therefore, DCM needs to conducted in a way that mirrors the desired culture for the care environment: with openness, sensitivity, and person centeredness.

DCM needs to be sensitively applied and to not lose sight of the core issue: One should treat others as one wishes to be treated. It is important to recognize how the initial introduction of DCM may disrupt a unit. The dominant culture in a unit may have developed over a long period of time, with its rewards and benefits for staff members. Suggested changes may be seen as unnecessary, intrusive, and threatening to the routines and style of a unit that seems to be running smoothly. Many professional care workers have never had any training in what is now called "dementia care." Their training sessions on dementia were likely brief, concentrating on medical aspects of the condition.

The introduction of a person-centered approach—and engagement, with its ideas and principles—will almost certainly affect how care workers view their roles. Following DCM training, one staff person said,

> *Since doing the training, I have realized that I am responsible for all of it. Not just when there's a break after tea. It's about how I take {a resident} down to breakfast and how I help her out of her chair, as well as what's available to help make life more fun at all those other odd times during the day.*

This sensitivity extends to every part of the care worker's duties and interactions. Workers become aware that the responsibility for the maintenance and enhancement of the social psychology (relationships, choice, interaction, occupation, and so on) lies with them and their co-workers. This has a profound effect on everyone for whom they care.

Preserving the dignity of people with dementia is important to many care workers and gives rise to discussion. A person-centered approach to dignity includes interpreting lessons from the person's life as well as being sensitive to family care workers. Buckland described this approach as *mindfulness*—that is, developing the ability to

> **Think** about what we know about the person, and about what they are expressing.
> **Feel** how we are feeling, and how it feels to be together.
> **Understand** how they might be feeling.
> **Do** respond to the person, enable them to make choices, support them in feeling valuable, encourage their "action" on their terms, treat them as a (close) friend, help them to feel "at home." (1995, p. 34)

FACTORS FOR DEMENTIA CARE MAPPING TO EFFECT CHANGE IN THE CULTURE OF CARE

Changes in the culture of care come about through a variety of means. For DCM to be a useful part of the change in culture, a number of factors are necessary. Support for the changes from the organization and those working within it is crucial.

Organizational Support

One necessary change in the culture of care is to give professional care workers support, encouragement, and the opportunity to engage in different work if they no longer have the passion or commitment required for working with people with dementia. Marshall remarked,

The challenge of caring for such patients is rarely recognized. It should imply highly trained, well supported staff with high status. The reality is that most staff are untrained, levels of agency staff are high, and management fails to provide the constant support and encouragement required. This results in burnt out staff who have neither the energy nor the drive to provide more than basic physical care. . . . Units that look after people with dementia need more investment—not just of money for staff and buildings, although these are important, but of time, skill, and energy. (2001, p. 411)

Addressing Challenges by Staff Teams

Challenges to mappers often sound similar to the following:

> *What does a nurse from a day center know about continuing care? What can you know? You've never worked here. You don't know our residents. You don't know what it's like working here. You don't understand the demands made on us.*

This challenge is to DCM per se. It says much about the anxiety and defensiveness of the care workers, but it also gives an opportunity to provide a meaningful response.

If care workers are to have confidence in DCM, it is important for staff teams to understand that specific experience is not necessary and that DCM can be an appropriate tool in most settings. Care workers must be given the opportunity to develop confidence in the ability of the mappers to empathize with them and the people for whom they care. The mappers need to demonstrate a willingness to listen to staff concerns about all aspects of their work. Mappers must be clear about their motives for mapping and that they are using DCM for the benefit of all in the unit—staff and people receiving care.

The implementation of DCM may be challenged for other reasons. For example, professional care workers may ask questions such as "What can we do when we have to respond to the demands of the ward round and the assessment processes, and when sedative drugs are prescribed?"

The desire to help the person with dementia and his or her family caregivers may compete with the apparent medicalization of the problems. Many health care workers would like to see changes in their wards and emphasis placed on outreach and community-based care. Some may have attended DCM training and may fully agree with its aims in principle. In the meantime, they know that hospitalization and sedation almost inevitably lead to loss of skills, disorientation, and decline in the person's ability to function independently in the future.

The DCM worker must be willing to address such concerns with the staff group and perhaps with managers and medical staff, too. Major aspects of the situations care workers face are likely to be beyond their control. DCM can help staff to see where they might make changes to their own practice and can also give them insights that enable them to challenge the ways in which they are expected to work.

Identifying and Addressing Conflicting Approaches to Care

Strong personalities among the staff can significantly influence the effectiveness of a DCM evaluation. For example, one or two care workers who are defensive and angry about the mapping can conspire to undermine the efforts of DCM workers. This point is illustrated in the following example:

> *Staff training had been provided, and the care unit of a large nursing facility was due for its second evaluation. One obstacle remained: gaining the residents' permission for the mapping. Staff believed that it was important to establish informed consent before a map took place. As relatives and family care workers rarely visited the unit, obtaining consent through family members was not a realistic possibility. At the next meeting between the staff and mappers, it became apparent that the manager was not in favor of the second evaluation. She believed that DCM was inappropriate for her unit.*

In this situation, the unit manager had been under pressure to embrace DCM. She and the staff had used all of the arguments they could think of to avoid having an evaluation take place. Person-centered care was at odds with what she thought "her" patients needed. She saw the unit's role as keeping the residents as safe and healthy as possible. At the same time, staff were burning out and becoming sick. The senior manager of the nursing facility subsequently admitted that this particular unit had problems, which she had hoped that DCM and training in person-centered care would address. In this context, staff suspected that DCM was being set up to do the senior management's job. This work involved changing the attitudes of staff, including the unit manager. The staff were still feeling marginalized, and the DCM implementation and results made them feel blamed as well.

Another example of a possible culture clash is the influence of medical staff and the way that doctors sometimes conduct their tasks. Challenges must be made regarding how the behavior of visiting doctors can affect residents and staff.

> *During a DCM evaluation, a doctor's round took place. The manager and several of the nurses were clearly expected to accompany the ward round, giving information about each person in turn. During the round,*

patients' activities were suspended, and music and the television were switched off. After the map, several of the nurses commented that they were not happy with the way that the doctors had spoken to patients and about patients in their presence, but the nurses had felt powerless to intervene.

Challenges must also be made regarding doctors' strong influence on how resources are allocated within the health care system. For years, the medical establishment made dementia care a low priority. This changed at the end of the 20th century, however, when various "cognitive enhancing" drugs were introduced. Measuring the effectiveness of these drugs increasingly centers on cognitive ability and decline rather than on well-being and way of life. Thus, challenging doctors' treatment of people with dementia challenges the whole medical model.

CONCLUSION

Hospital ward staff are likely to see the challenge of DCM as a challenge to their whole way of working. Duties and tasks—as well as uniforms, keys, medication, and handling visits from family care workers—are often questioned. These things are all part of the tradition of caring institutions. They constitute some of the barriers to being truly person-centered. Routines, uniforms, and locked doors help to maintain a sense of the importance of the work. Without them, would it be possible to tell the difference between those who have dementia ("Them") and those who deliver care ("Us")?

Those who work in social care settings have also developed their own set of obstacles to relating in a person-centered way. Like their health service colleagues, they have done this not in a deliberate attempt to be uncaring but in accordance with the traditions and culture of the services in which they find themselves. It takes a considerable effort in terms of learning, changing, and adapting to become truly person centered. If person-centered care is to flourish, then an organization must support its workers, giving them reasons other than keys and uniforms to value themselves.

DCM workers must be willing not only to challenge ways of working at a unit and organizational level, but also to support the efforts of staff to change and develop. DCM can help to effect change if mappers are aware of the various cultural influences in the setting in which DCM is proposed to work.

REFERENCES

Bell, J., & McGregor, I. (1994). Beyond the mask of conventional manners. *The Journal of Dementia Care, 2*(5), 18–19.

Bradford Dementia Group. (1997). *Evaluating dementia care: The DCM method* (7th ed.). Bradford, England: University of Bradford.

Buckland, S. (1995). Well-being, personality and residential care. In T. Kitwood & S. Benson, (Eds.), *The new culture of dementia care* (pp. 30–34). London: Hawker Publications.

Cassell. (1979). *Cassell's English dictionary*. London: Author.

Fleming, R. (1993). *Issues of assessment and design for longstay care*. Stirling, Scotland: University of Stirling, Dementia Services Centre.

Heller, R. (2001). *Evaluation of Woodcraft Folk Peer Education Project*. London: Woodcraft Folk.

Kitwood, T. (1997). *Dementia reconsidered: The person comes first*. Buckingham, England: Open University Press.

Kitwood, T., & Benson, S. (Eds.). (1995). *The new culture of dementia care*. London: Hawker Publications.

Marshall, M. (2001). The challenge of looking after people with dementia. *British Medical Journal, 323,* 410–411.

Merriam-Webster. (1997). *Merriam-Webster's collegiate dictionary* (10th ed.). Springfield, MA: Author.

Packer, T. (2000). Does person-centred care exist? *The Journal of Dementia Care, 8*(3), 19–21.

Pearsall, J. (Ed.). (2001). *New Oxford dictionary of English*. New York: Oxford University Press.

Waite, M. (Ed.). (1998). *The little Oxford dictionary* (Rev. 7th ed.). New York: Oxford University Press.

II

USING DEMENTIA CARE MAPPING TO IMPROVE CARE PRACTICE

4

A CRITICAL REFLECTION OF DEMENTIA CARE MAPPING IN GERMANY

CHRISTIAN MÜLLER-HERGL

Dementia Care Mapping (DCM) is strongly reminiscent of Grond's books and teachings in Germany (1996, 1997). Grond articulated a critique of dominant medical approaches, gave a sociopsychological perspective on dementia, and illustrated a determinate love for those who live with it. Therefore, the content of the DCM manual (Bradford Dementia Group, 1997) is not new to me, other than its combination of the humanistic approach (Morton, 1999) with the technical. Investing all knowledge about dementia care into an operational tool that measures well-being and, thereby, quality of care seems both fascinating and questionable. It is fascinating because learning how people with dementia feel is the holy grail of dementia care. So many practical problems originate from deficient understanding of the experience of people with dementia. The combination seemed questionable because it takes a long time for all therapists to reflect on and reliably use transference and countertransference. Can walking in the other's shoes be done so easily? Will measurements of their well-being not be a reflection or projection of the observers, of their understanding of dementia and ability to accept people who have it (Lawton et al., 2000)? This combination of fascination and doubt has never left me.

After briefly sketching the development of DCM in Germany, this chapter addresses the question of whether and how institutions providing dementia care can profit from the feedback process (see Phase 4 of Table 3 in the Introduction). The chapter concludes that formal feedback according to DCM makes sense only in institutions that have developed an advanced level of learning and communication. Also presented are the basics of an improved design for introducing DCM into practice.

DEMENTIA CARE AND
DEMENTIA CARE MAPPING IN GERMANY

There is widespread professional agreement in Germany concerning the adequacy of homogeneous dementia care units (i.e., the "segregative approach"), which concentrate exclusively on the needs of people with dementia and staff (Deutsche Alzheimer Gesellschaft, 2001). Special efforts are made to create an environment that "holds" or "contains" the person in a manner that reflects "atavistic" or "chaotic" themes of dementia. (For more information about atavistic themes— that is, the return to developmental themes in the beginning of the human species—see Eibel-Eibelsfeld, 1982, and Wojnar, 2001.) Nevertheless, until the beginning of the 21st century, only a small number of care homes in Germany made a sustained effort to change environment, staffing, and procedures. Most institutions are dominated by rigid procedures, through which work is done in the modus of getting finished or getting through what is regarded as essential or indispensable: control of the body, emotions, and behavior (e.g., see Darmann, 2000; Muthesius, 2000; Schopp et al., 2001). Individual needs are rarely met. In addition, interaction and communication generally are not person centered. Instead, they are characterized by mild and moderate forms of malignant social psychology (Kitwood, 1997) that are viewed as "natural" in essentially asymmetric relationships of high dependence. Most institutions and professional care workers are inclined to describe their practices as person centered and individualized. Evaluation is lacking, however, because methods of quality assurance that are specifically focused on dementia care are not available in Germany.

With the exception of Validation (Feil, 2002), the medical model of dementia reigns unchallenged in Germany (see Berger, 2001, and Förstl, 2001). Attacks on it are quickly ridiculed as being ideological. Dementia is reduced to challenging or disturbing behavior and efforts to control such behavior.

PRECONDITIONS FOR USING DEMENTIA CARE MAPPING

There are a number of lessons to be learned from the phases of introducing DCM in Germany.

Lessons from Phase 1

There was no grand design to introduce DCM in Germany. Instead, I adopted a step-by-step approach to investigate possible interest in the method. Well-established connections to some nursing facilities allowed me to prepare and run exemplar DCM courses and to accompany the introduction of DCM into the nursing facility system. These institutions were far advanced in terms of their organization. For example, staff, relatives, and volunteers participated in all major decisions and actions. Staff also had good communication and inter-action skills because of continuous external supervision. In addition, excellent internal cooperation existed because a process that valued consensus was in place. Furthermore, no additional problems impeded or blocked the introduction of DCM (e.g., rapid staff turnover, sudden staff shortages, sudden changes in management priorities).

Trainers and basic users mapped together in pairs. With time, they gained experience that informed their practice and use of the DCM method. One lesson learned was that it was best to map with only two mappers—one professional, one volunteer—at a time in a given area. In addition, it was learned that mapping results and feelings should be discussed among the mapper team before feedback. Designing and naming the function of a chief/lead mapper was also determined to be necessary. Finally, the need to coordinate all activities concerning mapping and to keep detailed records was established.

DCM follow-ups gave ample opportunity to discover and resolve imple-mentation difficulties. One essential result of this element was that the tradi-tional 3-day course in DCM did not enable people to apply the method. Follow-up sessions discussed issues such as coding problems and Personal Detractions (PDs), as observed through role play. Time was required to develop an action plan for the setting as well as for the newly trained mappers to accept and develop their roles. Such follow-up is necessary because DCM amounts to a major inter-vention in the nursing facility system and needs intensive support.

Lessons from Phase 2

A new phase started in January 2000. The Department for the Science of Nursing at the University of Witten/Herdecke organized a week-long course on dementia care. The course surveyed all of the approaches that were popu-lar at that time, devising strategies to research problems and to identify themes and challenges. Person-centered care and DCM seemed to strike a chord with most participants. The Kuratorium Deutsche Altershilfe (KDA—an organiza-tion similar to England's Age Concern) decided to support and sponsor the method in a sustained manner. As of 2002, DCM courses are organized throughout Germany. Several professionals (most of them Validation Therapy trainers or nurses) are preparing to become DCM trainers.

A certain degree of thought is invested into integrating DCM as part of a more comprehensive system of quality assurance and staff development. A shorter version is discussed for inspectors of Germany's medical service to provide them with information about what constitutes good practice and which practices require improvements. One lesson learned was that DCM is often used not so much for quality assurance but for the evaluation of certain interventions or the quality of a general environment of care. Some people use the instrument to identify environmental deficits and needs as well as training needs and staff requirements.

Initial findings also indicate problems in the internal organization of professional caregiving groups, which impede innovation and change of attitude. These groups seem to need prolonged, sustained support in their daily work for procedures to change.

Another lesson learned in Phase 2 was that specially arranged environments do not always make the desired difference for people with dementia. It is the care relationship that counts, those repeated efforts to give contact without necessarily doing something specific (i.e., having a staff presence).

In Germany, there is a marked contrast between interest in and application of DCM. There are difficulties in sustaining the application of the method. As the next section argues, DCM might contradict deeply ingrained attitudes of care staff who work in institutions.

THE DOGMA OF INSTITUTIONAL CARE

Observation and feedback—procedures central to the DCM approach—allow the method to refrain from intervention and mutual reflection (i.e., the "developmental loop"). Both observation and feedback are also central to ethnological discipline for the study of what Koch-Straube (1997) called the "alien" within "us." They represent on a symbolic level an anti-institutional affect: It is understanding that counts, not managing the "strange" behavior of people with dementia. Observation and feedback implicitly contradict the operative subtext of caring or nursing: Caring means intervening, judging, and acting quickly—all with the goal of keeping control. The DCM approach is apparently incompatible with institutional care. Unfortunately, many care workers in institutional environments intuitively realize this and, thus, strongly dislike DCM. They claim that it is too theoretical; does not tell one what to do; cannot be applied quickly and easily; and involves too much conflict, thought, and reflection. This sentiment reflects, in part, an unwillingness (perhaps an inability) to be personally involved and an urge not to disturb the status quo. Acceptable is that which can be introduced without too much change to the daily structure and defined, goal-directed care interventions. In such environments, every member of the team has to deliver his or her amount of defined "quantities" (i.e., people receiving care) for work approval. The following discussion of the logic of institutional care illustrates why this is so.

Nursing facilities are at the end of the service chain and constitute "negative containers" for all those who do not meet the leitmotif of modern care: the informed and enlightened older adult who lives in his or her own home, is taking care of him- or herself, and is therefore able live alone at home. People enter nursing homes out of dire necessity ("voluntary imprisonment") because they are essentially dependent on others ("emotional and physical incontinence"). Having this sort of dependence as an adult is an anathema and deeply contradicts self-ideals of what it is to be an individual. Highly dependent older people with dementia become society's "inner or hidden aliens" (i.e., shadows of societal ideals) and are outsourced to institutionalized care.

Negative containers tend to be totally institutional and to be closed worlds regarding perception, judgment, identity, and ritual. People living and working in them mirror each other, and both can be considered "inhabitants" with asymmetrical yet complementary roles. Staff have total responsibility for and power over residents' bodies and minds and (structurally) cannot be discharged of their active role, which usually results in the appropriation of others as objects of care. People who are living there tend to develop a "wrong self"—that is, to show excessive disabilities and resign from responsibility for their life ("the sister knows what is best"). Self-renunciation and passivity appear as substitute, negative identity: Without a future and totally at others' disposal, these people are left with their feelings (e.g., disgrace, fear, shame, loss) and are unable to advance to an objective perception of themselves.

Personal encounters are hardly possible, and functional contexts rule the day. Most significantly, it is impossible for people in both "inhabitant" groups to differentiate between their own wishes or desires and institutional reflexes, masks, or norms. For exmaple, the nurse does not want to bring Mrs. Clark to bed at 7:00 P.M., but she has to—or thinks she has to. Mrs. Clark has learned that the nurse will be happy if she willingly goes to bed and even seems to want to, although she never was one to go to bed early. Both lose subjectivity, experiential understanding, reflectiveness, and connectedness. There is good reason to surmise that institutional care cannot become person or interperson centered. Many professional care workers strive toward person-centered care within the operative logic of the "machine"—the purposeful, rational, systemic, and machine-like reactions and actions that are demanded of care work-

ers (e.g., mealtimes, nursing times, bedtimes, plans of all sorts) and create little islands that nourish professional self-ideals. In this context, care workers
may consider person-centered care creating special occasions to go the extra
mile: changing to the night shift to avoid the daily war between care workers
and care recipients about little things, going against the accepted social norms
or order in individual practice with residents in their bedrooms (e.g., lowering hygiene standards for a resident who fights against them, hugging a resident who asks for extra attention, letting a resident walk around naked). It is
generally left to the individual care worker or nurse how to practice personal
relations by concomitantly accepting the institutional definitions of life and
care (Dörner et al., 2001; Gröning, 2000; Gröning et al., 1995).

These small worlds develop their own subcultures and tend to define
everything from the outside as alien (e.g., physicians, relatives, inspectors, supervisors, teachers, researchers, mappers). The splitting of the inner and outer
worlds reflects the negative container concept from the inside out and sym-
bolizes the return of the repressed. Those from the outer world disturb established routines and rituals and the power connected with them. Routines and
rituals are survival routes in a complex situation of need that is difficult to
understand. They are, of course, necessary and maybe even a resource, but they
also embody attempts to control, civilize, or normalize the chaos of dementia
by regimentation, sanction, discipline, and the pathologization of behavior.
Even activities are delivered in the form of routines (e.g., singing and playing
games from 10:00 A.M. to 11:00 A.M.), and all individuals become part of "the
plan." Malignant social psychology is at the heart of the role and power construction of institutional care. The underlying theory is to save and reconsti-
tute social presentability of the clientele and to symbolically undo the "offense"
of dementia—it is not allowed to exist, to be lived out. It is fundamentally
unacceptable. Thus, these routines are not made and reconstituted every day
but are powers of destiny that nobody can really change.

The operative logic is the plan that organizes the day in an effective, purposeful, rational, and systemic way: nursing plans; meal plans; seating plans;
plans for breaks, communication, rest, sleep—you name it! The systemic element implies that every individual is a replaceable entity within the matrix.
The individual's point of view is excluded. In this setting, care workers perceive individuals' wishes that contradict institutional procedures or outright
rebellion as a personal affront. The system expects the patient to be a humble
participant, one who is happy about and grateful for what he or she receives,
does not make many demands, and resigns him- or herself to his or her fate.
The daily flow is disturbed by the individual. Individual attention impedes
the merciless efficiency and effectiveness and is judged as a beginner's prob-

lem. For example, a mapper who is giving feedback may focus on obvious PDs (e.g., fastening clothing protectors without communicating with the person). Replies from staff might be "Do you have practical experience?" or "Are you out of practice?"—thereby suggesting that questioning these humdrum affairs signals incompetence in practical matters. The plan, not the individual, stands in the middle of each organization. Rituals ban individuality.

Staff in institutional settings work on their own personal agendas by creating order and presentability. Every day, chaos overcomes the care setting. Symbolically undoing dementia helps the care worker deal with a complex situation. Straightening things out also allows staff to orientate themselves but not necessarily the people with dementia. In addition, addressing the chaos staves off certain staff fears: death, decay, shame, angst, disgust, losses, the shadow of one's own future, the trauma of having self-ideals disrupted. Caregiving seems to help undo these themes for the person and thereby stabilize his or her self-concept. These themes are also counteracted by an outer, fictitious order—an order that is constantly on the brink of collapse because of challenging behavior and its aggravation in the home context as well as limited resources. This results in little contact with people with dementia (e.g., "I'll be back in a minute," "I don't know right now," "Maybe tomorrow") or avoidance behavior (e.g., going outside for a cigarette break, ignoring apathetic residents). Contact is only possible and bearable in the modus of distance, such as contact with a resident while reaching out for the door handle. In Germany, the code for many nurses could be described as "sich hinter der pflege verstecken" ("hide behind nursing activities"). This behavior is a defense against the daily demand being made against one's own person: to share the lives of those who eat up one's energy. Highly dependent people can have power over another by being so dependent. In this context, particularly in combination with burnout, the care worker might be tempted to return the damaging feelings to the resident, which is the foundation of violence in institutional care settings. The constant and seemingly unreasonable demands on care workers result in burnout. This condition could actually be described as "coolout" because staff can become apathetic and insipid.

These suppressed emotions can cause professional care workers to oscillate between action (create order) and refusal (do not encounter residents in a person-centered way). The dialectic dilemma is solved by doing the necessary physical work, controlling the situation via routines and rituals, not asking for the meaning behind the routines, and falling back on a technical-functional form of contact that is the typical sign of proper service. In this context, service relates to people being treated as objects, not subjects. The result is quasi-intimacy, a quasi-family atmosphere that avoids real intimacy and contact.

That is, it prevents meeting the other person equally—on "eye-level"—and instead presents the mask, the role, the institutionalized reflex (Wolber, 1998).

Feelings reflect the inner logic of institutions better than their systemic plans. In Germany, the dominant perception of institutionalized staff has been connected with the myth of Sisyphus (Gröning, 1998) or, even more accurately, with the figuration of the abandoned mother with a hopeless child (Elias, 1976). That image is shared by all participants, and it informs and shapes the hidden agendas in nursing facilities (e.g., sick leave, job changes or leaving a job, difficulties with leadership) that reflect dissatisfaction with the working culture or expected behaviors. These actions are reflexes of depression on an institutional level. Naturally, such an unfavorable picture is something of an overgeneralization. Institutions differ greatly, and the previously described effects and phenomena might be minimal in smaller settings. Good leadership and a strong commitment to validating staff make some nursing homes better residences for people with dementia than their families' homes.

Nevertheless, based on my observations in various European countries, most institutions that provide care for people with dementia more or less demonstrate the phenomena described. As a result, observation, refraining from taking action, identifying with the individual, and reflecting while keeping shared goals in mind is and will be a strange, incommensurable factor within institutionalized systems of care. Many institution staff will not identify with a procedure that symbolically opens up small worlds to public eyes or that observes their actions from a third-person perspective—or from the perspective of the person with dementia. Mapping will not necessarily effect change; rather, staff may be tempted to resist further mappings. To that end, DCM underestimates the reluctance and resistance with which professional care workers meet the method.

INSTITUTIONAL CHALLENGES TO MAPPERS

Staff at institutions may find DCM interesting or even fascinating, but they are often at odds with permanent implementation of the DCM process (observation, evaluation, and implementation of action plans) within the existing order. DCM shares the fate of care planning and other rational instruments that attempt to individualize care and interrupt the flow. It has been my experience in staff supervision that if a mapper is from within the institution or the ward, then other staff typically avoid feedback that critiques practice.

When the Mapper Is a Staff Member

It may be that the person's role of care staff is incompatible with his or her mapper role. The mapper often does not confront colleagues with critical aspects of common practice; this symbolically takes the mapper out and above the group, and the group may be the person's only source of personal support in the caregiving role. People who provide care frequently are afraid of confrontations, look for security, and want orientation (just as many people with dementia need orientation and "leadership"). Mappers, especially inexperienced ones, may find it difficult to think through their observations, to focus on essential points, and to speak up and accept their new supervisory role. Often, there is no established practice for open communication about problems. The professional care field is not prepared for the kind of learning that DCM demands. This results in useless feedback and initiates the slow death of the method. Staff need comprehensive training in dementia care, communication skills, and skills for coping with their feelings after mapping feedback. As it stands, then, DCM is a tool for gerontological and psychiatric "elite," not a tool to encourage reflection among practitioners.

When the Mapper Is an Outsider

If mappers are from the outside, then staff often endure them passively—just as they endure staff shortages; training in care planning, kinesthetics, and Validation; or a new manager's latest whim. In the best cases, staff find the DCM results "interesting" and "stimulating." Without a comprehensive re-shuffling of service routines, focused training, changes in leadership, and—most important—work on team dynamics and the institutional feelings, most "interesting feedback" has little impact. Staff are unable to implement change because most must undergo further education in dementia care, as they do not have the power to change practice in the long term without the support of managers, policy makers, and so forth.

In addition, mappers from the outside come in the role of "experts." For staff who believe that their situation is hopeless, external experts are often aliens (who, like managers, do not understand or care about existing team dynamics) or redeemers (who should tell staff what to do). Both roles are counterproductive, as they prevent discovering and developing one's own expertise and responsibility. The outside expert needs an attitude of contact *with* distance (i.e., a supervisory role).

Furthermore, external specialists are expensive and employed only for baseline mappings or for evaluations of specific interventions. A long-standing developmental companionship is rarely envisioned, but learning processes that change attitudes take years. It is often the case, however, that little steps are quickly swallowed by the old system in the face of the first crisis. Under stress, one returns to the old pattern—and stress is universal in geriatric care!

Summary

Challenges to mappers, as well as institutional dogma, cast doubt on whether institutions can possibly profit from DCM. Mapping and feedback alone have little chance to change and interrupt the flow of care. Changes in care and in the implementation of DCM are necessary if the method is to be effective.

IMPROVED DESIGN FOR
IMPLEMENTING DEMENTIA CARE MAPPING

Key elements are needed for a culture of change. First, establish a basic understanding of what caring for people with dementia implies and demands. Second, require a continuous reflection of care practice in case work. Third, enact a system of support and role models for change agents (e.g., qualified dementia care workers). Fourth, form an agreement among management, change agents, and staff about priorities and procedures. Finally, integrate changes in the daily work structure (Müller-Hergl, 2000). When all of these aspects are fully covered, they amount to thorough education and skill development in dementia care.

The German Ministry of Health (BMG) projected a DCM-supported regional quality development program. This program separately examined the potential of three central change aspects:

1. Exploring the sociopsychological theory of dementia and the principles of positive person work (i.e., concept formation)

2. Ensuring awareness of and empathy for people with dementia (i.e., hermeneutical understanding and case work)

3. Giving feedback to teams and developing action plans

From a broad base of elementary qualification for all staff (Aspect 1), some people become mappers (Aspect 3) and, in regional conferences, help to identify best practices in dementia care. This defined practice becomes the empirical basis for evaluating innovation in the dementia care field. Aspect 1 can be used for a wide variety of purposes. It is not necessarily connected with DCM; for example, it could just as well be used for management and leadership issues in dementia care. There are academic ways or workshop procedures to identify and discuss development and teaching requirements.

In the BMG's DCM program, Aspect 1 is the cornerstone of a seminar that provides all staff with basic information about dementia care. This is followed by training in integrative Validation, kinesthetics, sensory stimulation, and reminiscence, as well as training in nonverbal body communication (e.g., body mimicry, tonic dialogue). The idea is that whether professionals or not, most staff have not received a basic training for working with older people who have special sociopsychological needs. Accordingly, all new members of staff have to go through this training within their first year of work.

Disciplining empathy and awareness—for example, through the DCM coding system—can be used for a variety of purposes: within the primary education for medical professionals, for the education of mental health nurses, for home inspectors, or for researchers. Slipping into another person's shoes is susceptible to projection, however, particularly for Behaviour Category Codes (BCCs) such as C (Cool—withdrawn behavior). Passivity and "vegetative" behavior in people with dementia are not well understood. The connected validity and reliability problems can be tackled best if using these codes presupposes the mapper's close observation of him- or herself (i.e., reactive observation or countertransference) and extended training in reading the emotional meaning of facial and motor expressions and body language (Lawton et al., 2000). This implies learning to distinguish the answers to four questions:

1. What do I actually see?

2. What do I feel and what are my inner pictures?

3. What does it remind me of (in my own history)?

4. How do I interpret the situation?

People have to learn in a disciplined way to distinguish observation and interpretation; thereby, they acquire skills that are normally applied in ethnological studies. Understanding dementia involves reflecting on body language—that is, "tuning in" to another person through nonverbal means only. Tuning in involves observing muscle tone, breathing, rhythm of movement, position in the room, eye contact, and gestures—first for oneself and then for the other person observed. One has to learn how emotions and moods are transported through one's own body language and that of a training group before one can reliably discern the range of feelings associated with, for example, apathy. Working on nonverbal body language disciplines one's observations and is a way to distinguish observation from interpretation. Learning to mimic another person's movements, gestures, sounds, and breathing enables the observer to make educated guesses concerning well-being.

In the BMG project, training to use the DCM coding system is integrated in learning about body language. Observers proceed from basic training (Aspect 1), follow their coded observations (Aspect 2), and meet in supervised groups (Aspect 3). Role-playing and discussion are used to check the distinction between observation and interpretation. Individual emotions will come to the surface. People who are learning to observe in a disciplined way work on their own sensibility and sensitivity without the stress of giving feedback to a team. The most important intervention on this level is the change that observation and reflection trigger in professional staff. Trainers use defined evaluation procedures to identify the change within the working teams. These experienced trainers and supervisors accompany training groups for a year.

Only a small, select number of observers decide to give formal feedback about their external perspective (Aspect 3). The validity of the data processing in the seventh edition of the DCM manual (Bradford Dementia Group, 1997) is questionable (see Chapter 2 of this book for a fuller discussion). Thus, the key task is training observers to work through and reflect on their maps in a phenomenological and hermeneutical fashion—that is, using central qualitative statements and focusing on aspects that staff would find authentic because they are

• Detailed and precise

• Relevant and to the point

• Empathetic and caring

• Oriented to manageable change and development

After mapping, observers meet in their groups, share their feelings, and reflect on their observations. Accompanied by supervisors or experienced trainers, participants prepare feedback sessions through role play. Obviously, the ability to accept one's observations, defend them before a group, and come to a common understanding and plan is a fundamental skill in caregiving. DCM is used to work on these basic skills.

Mappers learn to shape their role and to integrate it into their general job profile. In the beginning, they give rudimentary feedback. After conducting some reflective mappings, they start to develop action plans with the team. Gradually, they learn to identify team dynamics and how to gear their feedback according to what a team can take.

For at least 3 years, one of the mappers serves as moderator of the mapping process. This person is in close contact with management to coordinate mappings, feedback, and action plans. Every team is obliged to develop action plans and to share them with management.

Kitwood (1997) envisioned a "reflective practitioner" in dementia care. Reflection must be learned by both sides: by the staff as a genuine chance to develop and by mappers to advance the staff's capacity for development. The use of DCM as a feedback instrument is the result of a process that takes time and energy. Factors that obviously shape this process are education, an internal support system for mappers, and external supervision. Useful feedback presupposes that the mapper is mature, professional, objective, and open to the perspectives of others. Until the implementation of the BMG's program, most nursing facility staff had difficulty cultivating all of these qualities without substantial and sustained support from the outside.

CONCLUSION

This chapter asserts that observation and feedback contradict the logic behind thought and action within institutional care in Germany. Thus, DCM can only be applied in institutions that are far advanced in their learning process. For competent application of the tool, far more is needed than what is taught in the 3-day course. Beginning mappers should only give brief feedback on their observations. Giving feedback requires the skills 1) to analyze whether an institution is ready for DCM and 2) to develop, with the team, a reasonable action plan. People doing those two things should have extra training.

Over and above the already mentioned points, the following aspects must be integrated into DCM implementation:

- An analysis of environmental factors, particularly choices and options available to staff

- An analysis and description of staff attitudes toward and knowledge about the people with dementia

- The training status of staff

- Interviews with staff and people who have dementia

- Field notes in the style of ethnological studies

- An analysis and description of management and leadership in gerontopsychiatric work

- An awareness of rituals and routines in the setting

Finally, several follow-ups and mapper supervision sessions should accompany DCM implementation. DCM is a major intervention for an institution and needs careful preparation and support.

REFERENCES

Berger, H. (2001). Ein Perspektivenwechsel in der Psychiatrie. *Dr. med. Mabuse*, 26–129.
Bradford Dementia Group. (1997). *Evaluating dementia care: The DCM method* (7th ed.). Bradford, England: University of Bradford.

Darmann, I. (2000). Anforderungen der Berufswirklichkeit an die kommunikative Kompetenz von Pflegekräften. *Pflege,* 13–4.

Deutsche Alzheimer Gesellschaft. (2001). *Stationäre versorgung von Alzheimer-patienten.* Leitfaden für den Gesellschaft Umgang mit demenzkranken Menschen, Berlin.

Dörner, K. et al. (2001). Für eine Auflösung der Heime: Anforderung an den Deutschen Bundestag, eine Kommission zur "Enquete der Heime" einzusetzen. *Dr. med. Mabuse,* 26–133.

Eibel-Eibelsfeld, I. (1982). Liebe und Hass: Zur Naturgeschichte elementarer Verhaltensweisen München.

Elias, N. (1976). Der Prozeß der Zivilisation, Frankfurt, Bd.I.

Feil, N. (2002). *The Validation breakthrough: Simple techniques for communicating with people with "Alzheimer's-type dementia"* (2nd ed.). Baltimore: Health Professions Press.

Förstl, H. (2001). *Demenzen in theorie und praxis.* Berlin.

Grond, E. (1996). *Praxis der Psychischen Altenpflege.* Freiburg.

Grond, E. (1997). *Altenpflege als Beziehungspflege.* Hagen.

Gröning, K. (1998). *Entweihung und Scham: Grenzsituationen in der Pflege alter Menschen.* Frankfurt.

Gröning, K. (2000). Institutionelle Mindestanforderungen bei der Pflege von Dementen. In P. Tackenberg et al. (Eds.), *Demenz und Pflege.* Frankfurt.

Gröning, K. et al. (1995). *Institutionsgeschichten, institutionsanalysen: Sozialwissenschaftliche Einmischungen in Etagen und Schichten ihrer Regelwerke.* Tübingen.

Kitwood, T. (1997). *Dementia reconsidered. The person comes first.* Buckinhgam, England: Open University Press.

Koch-Straube, U. (1997). *Fremde Welt Pflegeheim: Eine ethnologische studie.* Bern.

Lawton, M.P. et al. (2000). Emotion in people with dementia: A way of comprehending their preferences and aversions. In P.M. Lawton & R.L. Rubinstein (Eds.), *Interventions in dementia care.* New York: Springer Publishing Co.

Morton, I. (1999). Person-centred approaches to dementia care.

Müller-Hergl, C. (2000). Personen-Programme-Prozeduren: Perspektiven einer Weiterbildung für Demenzpflege und Gerontopsychiatrie im Praxisverbund. In P. Tackenberg et al. (Eds.), *Demenz und pflege.* Frankfurt.

Muthesius, D. (2000). Musiktherapie in der Stationären Altenpflege. *Dr. med. Mabuse,* 25–127.

Schopp, A., et al. (2001). Autonomie, Privatheit und die Umsetzung des Prinzips der "informierten Zustimmung" im Zusammenhang mit pflegerischen Interventionen aus der Perspektive des älteren Menschen. *Pflege,* 14–1.

Teising, M. (Ed.). Altern (1998). *Äußere realität, innere wirklichkeiten.* Opladen/Wiesbaden.

Wojnar, J. (2001). Demenzkranke verstehen. In P. Dürrmann (Ed.), *Besondere stationäre Dementenbetreuung.* Hanover.

Wolber, E. (1998). Von der ritualisierten Distanz in Pflegepraxis und Pflegetheorie zu einer Begegnung auf Augenhöhe. *Pflege,* 11–3.

5

USING DEMENTIA CARE
MAPPING DATA FOR
CARE PLANNING
PURPOSES

ANTHEA INNES

Conducting a Dementia Care Mapping (DCM) evaluation generates a wealth of data. The four coding frames alone produce much information for individuals observed and the client group as whole. In addition, general observations of the setting, which are similar to ethnographic observations (Hammersley & Atkinson, 1995), are recorded as basic notes to provide further information and the potential to engender additional ideas for improvement and development of a care setting. (See Chapter 3 for more information about general observations.) This chapter considers how data collected under the four coding frames can be used to develop care plans for individuals with dementia and for the complete client group. Furthermore, examples of utilizing ethnographic observations to develop care are provided. The chapter concludes with an outline of the possibilities offered by creating care plans that draw on life history information to complement DCM data.

PRACTICAL USES OF DEMENTIA CARE MAPPING

Various practical applications of DCM stem from its four coding frames: Behaviour Category Coding (BCC), Well- and Ill-Being (WIB), Personal Detractions (PDs), and Positive Event Records (PERs). These coding frames are detailed in the following subsections.

Behaviour Category Codes

One strength of DCM is the range of experiences captured within the BCC framework. The activities or behaviors of each person observed provide a rich resource for staff teams to consider the pattern of the care day as well as the level of input that each individual with dementia receives or requires from paid care workers and others. Discussion of BCC data allows a succinct summary of the period observed and offers opportunities for the team to consider the level of input that an individual may require to enhance his or her well-being.

Presenting BCC data graphically provides a means for staff to discuss why certain behavior categories are absent, high, or low for an individual or for all individuals observed. Figure 5.1 provides an example. In this sample, low levels of activities—such as expressive (E), handicraft (H), and intellectual activities (I)—would be discussed. Record would be made of staff suggestions for introducing activities that individuals may enjoy, with the intent of enhancing their well-being. Low levels of distress (D) and instances in which staff did not respond to individuals (U) might also be discussed, highlighting strategies that staff adopt to avoid or deal sensitively with individuals' distress. The presence of high levels of distress (D) gives the staff team an opportunity to consider why this may be and how they can address difficult situations. (See Table 2 in the Introduction for a complete explanation of the codes given beneath Figure 5.1.)

Well-Being and Ill-Being

WIB data can also be presented graphically. This provides the staff group with an overview of the time that individuals or the client group spent in each of the six WIB bands. (See Table 2 in the Introduction for a complete explanation of WIB codes.) Figure 5.2 illustrates WIB data for a group. In this sample, WIB data often peaks at the +1 level. The data offer staff the opportunity to explore why there were little or no +3 or +5 levels of well-being and how to address this absence. The BCC data could then be used with WIB data to enable the staff group to consider whether, for example,

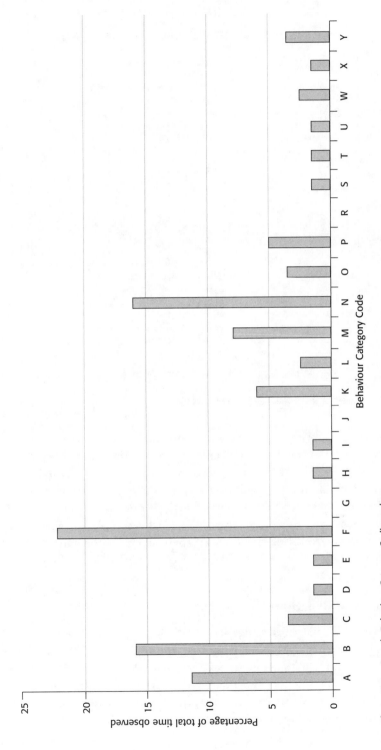

Figure 5.1. Sample Behaviour Category Coding values.

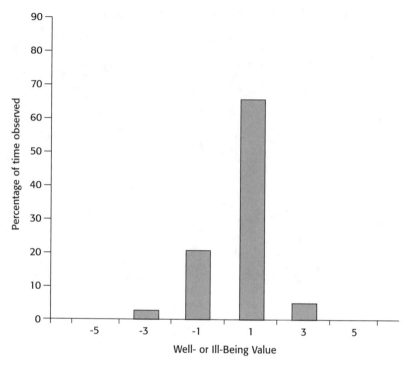

Figure 5.2.   Well- and Ill-Being (WIB) Codes for a group.

more one-to-one interactions would benefit individuals, activities such as crossword puzzles would be popular, or mealtime experiences could be improved. Individual WIB graphs can also be computed. If an individual is shown to have high levels of time in the −3 or −5 bands, then staff can begin focusing their attention on how to improve the person's well-being or to provide assistance and reassurance to an individual who may, for instance, be extremely anxious. It is important to compute graphs for the individual and for the group, as the group profile could disguise high levels of ill-being for an individual.

Personal Detractions

Kitwood (1997) identified categories of PDs as examples of malignant social psychology. Role-playing examples of observed instances of PDs can be very effective, resulting in team discussions of ways to reduce PDs. Individual Care Summaries, which are included in a report to the staff team, document the analysis of data as well as staff and observer comments on the care day. This information provides an initial springboard for developing a care plan for a person with dementia. PDs noted in the Individual Care Summary can be considered in relation to the activities and well-being of the person with dementia, allowing a holistic vision of a care plan to emerge. See Figure 5.3 for a sample Individual Care Summary.

Positive Event Records

The positive event coding frame outlined in the seventh edition of the DCM manual (Bradford Dementia Group, 1997) is the least developed DCM coding frame. Kitwood (1997) expanded on the concept with a discussion of *positive person work*. This framework has much to offer the dementia care practitioner, manager, policy maker (at the organizational level), and action researcher. One of DCM's underlying principles is the desire to improve and develop care practices and the lives of people with dementia. (See Chapter 1 for a discussion of DCM's theoretical origins.) Thus, for those involved in the care setting, positive person work offers indicators of good practice and areas worthy of further consideration. Developing this framework is a newer area of study (see Chapter 6). For example, Kasayka, Hatfield, and Innes (2001) included the perspectives of music, dance, and art therapists in an exploration of the relationship between healing art therapies and the full range of positive person work concepts—recognition, negotiation, collaboration, play, timalation (directly engaging the senses), relaxation, validation, holding, giving, facilitation, creation, and celebration. Such an approach could be developed for the care offered by other care workers, nurses, social workers, and occupational therapists. This approach would provide not only a record of the positive event (see Figure 5.4 for an example) but also an indication for the care worker of how his or her existing skills and professional ideology affect the well-being of individuals with dementia.

DRAWING INFERENCES FOR CARE PLANNING

The examples of data presented in Figures 5.1, 5.2, 5.3, and 5.4 illustrate the detailed information that can be presented for the group and for each person with dementia observed. These data highlight the overall well-being, behavior and activities patterns, and specific examples of when people with dementia experienced a PD (with the potential to reduce well-being) or a positive event (with the potential to increase well-being). Therefore, the team has a starting point for developing care plans that focus on the psychosocial aspects of care provision. This information is further complemented by the ethnographic observations that many mappers record. For example, key issues

Individual Care Summary

Place: <u>Sunnyvale Court</u>　　　　　　Date: <u>December 1</u>

Participant: <u>Vincent</u>　　　　　　Mapping period: <u>9.00 A.M.–3.00 P.M.</u>

Well- or Ill-Being (WIB) value profile

WIB value	−5	−3	−1	+1	+3	+5
Percentage of time observed	N/A	2	16	80	2	N/A

Highest scores in Behaviour Category Coding (BCC)

BCC	A	B	K	T	F
Percentage of time observed	6	29	33	8	16

Comments on care and quality of life:

Vincent kept himself going in many respects. He walked around the building and the garden, and he spent time shutting windows and doors and looking in cupboards. He asked for cigarettes and drinks, although these requests were not always noticed. He sometimes intruded on other residents' space, but this action could have been reduced if Vincent had more activities to keep him happily occupied. It appeared that he was seeking contact with others. He enjoyed his meals, but it seemed that he could do with second helpings, as he was still hungry and tried to take food from other residents' plates.

Comments on personal detractions:

Mild ignoring: On numerous occasions, Vincent asked for a cigarette but was given no response.

Mild invalidation: His perspective was overlooked in one instance. When Vincent described others in the room as "sleeping," care staff tried to get him to accept that those individuals were watching television, not sleeping.

Moderate outpacing: There was one incident of outpacing. Staff tried to hurry Vincent to the toilet, and this distressed him.

General comments:

Vincent tidied up after he ate, so perhaps more could be made of this action to include him in clearing tables or wiping them. More encouragement to sing and play the piano may help maintain and improve Vincent's well-being, as he clearly enjoys both activities. After lunch may be the best time to try to spend some time with Vincent, as he appeared to have more energy after eating. He may like spending time on his own. Yet, the way that Vincent looked at others who were talking or playing cards together suggests that he may be happy with others at times.

Figure 5.3.　Sample Individual Care Summary.

Positive Event Record

Time: Regular intervals throughout the care day

Participant: Rosemary

Description of positive event: Rosemary appeared to be an extremely anxious woman. Her partial blindness contributed to her need for reassurance and verbal explanations of who was near her and what was going on. The staff team displayed sensitivity and skill in their consistent offers of reassurance through speech and touch. Other clients sitting in the same area were encouraged to respond to Rosemary, leading to many short but lively exchanges and discussions among the client group as whole.

Significance: The staff team facilitated interactions between Rosemary and other residents, leading to increased well-being for everyone sitting in the lounge. Staff recognized Rosemary's anxiety, and their support often resulted in Rosemary visibly relaxing and stating, "I feel better now. Thanks, Dear."

Figure 5.4. Sample Positive Event Record.

emerging from observations of the setting in its entirety can be included in the evaluation report. Common issues that arise from mapping are

- Although it is understandable that staff are sometimes distracted by other client demands, all clients need regular fluids. This point is particularly important given the findings of the *Food for Thought* report (Alzheimer's Society, 2000), which suggested that people with dementia are not given enough to drink in hospitals or care homes.

- Television and radio are used inappropriately (sometimes both are on at the same time in the same room). This situation creates a noisy and disorientating environment and reduces the potential for meaningful communication (Goldsmith, 1996).

- Low levels of activities are offered for the group. Often, a few residents who are more vocal, mobile, and able (physically or cognitively) benefit from activities regularly while residents who are less vocal, mobile, and able are excluded. Based on the WIB coding frame, this exclusion results in an observable impact on the well-being of the excluded individuals.

The specific points that are raised for individuals can thus be considered in relation to general observations of the care setting. This comparison can result in, for instance, placing greater attention on meal and drink times to ensure that individuals do not become dehydrated and, potentially, more confused. Consideration of the physical environment may examine the use of media as a substitute for care worker attention and, in turn, the possibility that a noisy, disorientating environment raises anxiety and stress levels for both clients and care workers. The location of activities can also be considered. An alternative, larger space could be used to allow those who do not participate directly to observe (i.e., to include passive participants). The range of offered activities can also be considered, perhaps leading to a recognition that staff require further development opportunities. (See Chapter 6 for a discussion of staff training and development needs that arise from DCM.)

DEMENTIA CARE MAPPING, LIFE HISTORY, AND CARE PLANNING

After initial observations of the care setting, mappers often anecdotally comment on care workers' apparent lack of awareness regarding the life history of the observed individuals. Discussions with the staff in feedback sessions (see Phase 4 of Table 3 in the Introduction) often contradict this impression. A care worker, particularly one with special responsibility for the person with dementia (e.g., the individual's key worker), often carries a wealth of information about the individual. Unfortunately, this information is not always shared with other members of the care team. When a staff member leaves the care setting, the information that he or she has accumulated over time often leaves with him or her. This situation suggests a need for formal life history work within care settings (Murphy, 1994), with information recorded in life history books, boxes, or pictures or simply in a section of a care plan. The value of life history work in providing individualized care has been documented (Pietrukowicz & Johnson, 1991). In addition, some education programs provide a means of encouraging staff to begin developing life history work—an aspect of training that staff appear to value and enjoy (Innes, 2001). Care plans offer the opportunity for staff to draw on life history material. Skill is required, however, in translating often basic comments. Say that an individual with dementia "enjoys music." A staff member who is interested in making this a regular activity for the individual might learn that "enjoys music" means "enjoys *live* music" rather than videotapes or audiotapes. "Enjoys live music" might be further developed to "enjoys *dancing to* live music" and so forth, until a comprehensive approach to accommodating this preference is established within the care plan.

It can be difficult for care workers to gather life history information if the person's relatives live at a distance or if the person has no known living relatives. Patience and perseverance may be required to develop and alter a care plan that builds on current preferences, which may have changed considerably over time or with the progression of the individual's dementia.

A further challenge for staff is incorporating life history information and the DCM observations discussed in DCM feedback sessions into tangible actions and realistic goals. Constraints will be present: Financial resources, staff time, and the setting's physical environment and geographical location may make it difficult to respond to an individual's preferences. For example, an individual who once enjoyed regular walks along the beach may now live in a care setting that is near family members but is a 2-day journey to a beach. Yet, alternatives can be explored: walks by a river or a lake or in another pleasant outdoor area, such as a park or the woods. Frequently providing favorite meals, snacks, or drinks may also be difficult within a limited budget or diet (e.g., for a person with diabetes who also has a sweet tooth). Occasionally providing a small amount of the preferred item may be a compromise rather than the ideal, but it is a more realistic goal for the staff team.

DCM data can play a role in goal setting. Addressing BCC results may be a way to set realistic goals, such as reducing unattended distress (U) or slightly increasing interactions (A). Increasing the percent of time spent in +3 or +5 bands of well-being can be more challenging. An individual may participate in a greater range of BCC activities, but his or her well-being may only increase to the +1 band. Similarly, attempts to introduce positive events may fail for a variety of reasons: The person with dementia may be tired, ill, or not responding in the way that staff had hoped. Small targets are therefore necessary, and these may involve maintaining the present level of well-being and behavior categories and the occasional positive event. The staff group may set team targets to reduce the number of PDs, such as trying to avoid infantilization (speaking to or treating a resident as though he or she were a child).

CONCLUSION

DCM data can provide indicators for areas of care that need improvement and further development for individual members of staff and for the care setting as a whole. These changes can be fed into individual care plans and programs offered in the setting. Doing so effectively requires knowledge of each individual's life history. Goal planning and actions will succeed only if they are attainable and realistic. Increasing, maintaining, and enhancing well-being is at the heart of person-centered care (Kitwood, 1997); however, targets for increasing well-being or eliminating PDs may be unrealistic and ultimately impossible to achieve. Therefore, DCM coding frames should not be used as indicators and goals for improvement in isolation from other factors that influence care and well-being. Rather, DCM data should be used to *inform* care planning.

REFERENCES

Alzheimer's Society. (2000). *Food for thought*. London: Author.

Bradford Dementia Group. (1997). *Evaluating dementia care: The DCM method* (7th ed.). Bradford, England: University of Bradford.

Goldsmith, M. (1996). *Hearing the voice of people with dementia: Opportunities and obstacles*. London: Jessica Kingsley Publishers.

Hammersley, M., & Atkinson, P. (1995). *Ethnography: Principles in practice*. London: Routledge.

Innes, A. (2001). Student centred learning and person centred dementia care. *Education and Ageing, 16*(2), 229–252.

Kasayka, R.E., Hatfield, K., & Innes, A. (2001). Conclusion. In A. Innes & K. Hatfield (Eds.), *Healing arts therapies and person-centred dementia care* (pp. 113–121). London: Jessica Kingsley Publishers.

Kitwood, T. (1997). *Dementia reconsidered: The person comes first*. Buckingham, England: Open University Press.

Murphy, C. (1994). *It started with a sea shell*. Stirling, Scotland: Dementia Services Development Centre.

Pietrukowicz, M., & Johnson, M. (1991). Using life histories to individualize care. *Gerontologist, 31*(1), 102–106.

6

DEMENTIA CARE
MAPPING AND
STAFF DEVELOPMENT

MARIA SCURFIELD-WALTON

Numerous publications have indicated the value of Dementia Care Mapping (DCM) as a quality assurance mechanism that enables improvements in the quality of care of people with dementia (Brooker, Forster, Banner, Payne, & Jackson, 1998; Buckland, 1995; Williams & Rees, 1997). Although endorsing these values, this chapter argues that DCM alone will not bring about the changes in practice that are required to develop a person-centered dementia care culture. The chapter describes the experiences of introducing DCM into practice within a psychiatric hospital and the subsequent systematic approach to creating a strategy for staff development and practice development. In addition, the chapter explores how these staff and practice development initiatives have been implemented and the subsequent impact on person-centered care practices for patients, staff, and practice. (Key outcomes of these initiatives are presented in Table 6.1.)

INTRODUCTION OF DEMENTIA CARE MAPPING

In 1995, the Mental Health in Old Age Directorate at England's South of Tyne and Wearside National Health Service Trust (hereafter called "the Trust") intro-

Table 6.1. Key outcomes following the implementation of Dementia Care Mapping (DCM) within a practice development and staff development strategy at the Trust

Patient perspective	Practice perspective	Staff perspective
A 4-year audit of DCM evaluations has indicated the following outcomes:	Action planning guidelines focus on a team's strengths and the development of needs following DCM evaluations.	Staff questionnaires indicate a much more positive attitude toward DCM and its potential for improving care improvements.
• Occupational and sensory needs are being addressed.	The significance of positive events has led to sharing skills and valuing staff.	Staff are more demanding regarding the needs of their patients and themselves, and there is a greater sense of team cohesion.
• Many sensory and activity projects have developed.	More emphasis is placed on the structured day, based on residents' lifestyles and occupational needs.	Clinical supervision has provided opportunities for skill development, practice development, and personal growth.
• The introduction of life stories has led to a deeper understanding of the resident as a person and has influenced nurse–resident interpersonal relationships.	Mealtimes, which were once chaotic, are now calm and organized and reflect patient choices and preferences.	Positive person work has provided a framework for staff development.
• Well- and Ill-Being profiles are being used to evaluate activity programs.	Awareness of the use of the environment, particularly physical space, has increased significantly.	Staff are much more aware of the necessity for emotional and psychological care.
• Opportunities have increased for including people with dementia in decisions about their care.	The following have been established: 1) a major multidisciplinary review of care, including representatives from all clinical areas, and 2) a directorate philosophy of care, along with directorate values and beliefs.	Staff are utilizing creative methods to explore the experience of dementia.
• Personal detractions have decreased significantly.		Staff are developing skills in listening to the voices of people with dementia; they use a range of communication strategies (e.g., verbal, nonverbal, sensory, music, reminiscence) and resolution techniques.

duced DCM as a key quality assurance method. Initially, three staff members from this directorate, two staff nurses, and an enrolled nurse were selected for basic DCM training. The rationale for training this staff, as opposed to more senior clinicians, was to enhance the clinical credibility of the method and to influence positive changes in care practice. Following successful completion of the course, the enthusiastic mappers began giving presentations to co-workers about the DCM method. These presentations were intended to raise awareness about DCM and its potential impact on the quality of patient care, to inform staff of the methodology, and to prepare staff for DCM evaluations of clinical areas.

Initial responses from some nursing staff at the Trust were fairly negative; they found it difficult to relate DCM to improvements in patient care and felt threatened by the evaluation method and the introduction of a relatively new concept. In addition, not all staff were familiar with the person-centered care practices, which were also relatively new. Some nurses responded positively, however, as did other members of the multidisciplinary team, members of the quality department, line managers, and purchasers. This acceptance assisted in driving the initiative forward.

An extensive range of presentations was facilitated prior to the Trust's first map, which took place in a continuing care ward. Following the DCM evaluation, feedback presentations with the ward team were organized. One aim of this feedback was to give the ward team ownership of the information so it could plan improvements in patient care. Yet, some staff found great difficulty in accepting the feedback and perceived it as criticism of their caregiving (see Chapter 4 for further discussion of this issue). These staff members dwelt on the negative aspects of the feedback, particularly the Personal Detractions (PDs) that were highlighted. Some staff were very defensive and unwilling to acknowledge the effect of PDs on patients' well-being. Throughout the feedback session, the staff team was also reluctant to acknowledge any positive effects of the evaluation. The ward team focused their anger on the mappers, making the mappers feel alienated, isolated, and increasingly vulnerable.

This experience raised important issues of maintaining the well-being of both the mappers and the clinical staff. During this time, the mappers sought informal support from colleagues—both mappers and nonmappers. On reflection, it was assumed that clinical staff would immediately embrace person-centered care practices, including DCM; however, the outcome of the first evaluation showed that this was not the case.

DEVELOPING A NEW STRATEGY

To address the previously described issues, a strategy was formulated that included operational, practice development, and staff development initiatives.

DCM evaluations were postponed for a year to concentrate on implementing the strategy at the Trust.

Operational Issues

It was agreed that to provide support, more mappers would be trained. In addition, the range of mappers would be widened to include clinical leaders, managers, and educators. After this round of training, it became clear that there was a need to examine how the team was to move forward and to develop standards of practice in relation to DCM. It also became apparent that regular group meetings for mappers would be required to offer support, discuss professional and operational issues, plan maps, and develop personally. As a result, a DCM special interest group was established to explore operational, professional, and developmental issues relating to mapping. The group met each month for $1\frac{1}{2}$ hours.

At its inaugural meeting, the group agreed on its points of reference. Work began on an operational policy for DCM, which was distributed to ward managers for discussion with their teams. This policy also ensured a consistent approach for all mappers. To enhance coordination and consistency, a presentation package for delivery to clinical areas was developed alongside a data collection pack for the mappers. As part of the presentation pack, questionnaires were developed to assess the attitudes and opinions of clinical staff regarding DCM.

Training Program for Staff Development

Over a period of time, person-centered care training was enacted for all grades of staff. This was initially facilitated in house and included mappers and external experts (members of the Bradford Dementia Group and other experts in the dementia field). Since 2000, practice development nurses and mappers have facilitated a rolling training program that gives an overview of person-centered care principles and focuses on challenges in practice. Training concentrates on skill development, particularly in communication, listening to people with dementia, and care planning.

To meet the needs of clinicians, assessment, interventions, and evaluation of challenging behavior are also included. The program concludes with a workshop on person-centered approaches for staff. In fact, the overall training is facilitated by a mostly workshop format, with an emphasis on reflection and interaction. A wide range of training materials are also utilized throughout the program (e.g., Journal of Dementia Care, 1996–1997; Killick, 1997; Loveday & Kitwood, 1998).

Evaluation of the training program has yielded positive responses from staff, who indicated that focusing on skill development and providing opportunities for staff to reflect and debate their practice influenced their development. The biggest impact on staff continues to be the use of experiential learning, including role playing, which attempts to demonstrate the consequences of PDs and the influences of positive person work for the person with dementia.

Practice Development

In 2001, a personal and practice development plan was incorporated into the program. Using a structured outline as a guide, staff are expected to develop a plan regarding an aspect of the training that they want to develop into their own practice area. Following the training program, staff have approximately 2–3 months to complete their plan, with support and guidance from their line manager and practice development nurse. Then, staff meet as a group and present their plans, implementation strategies, and evaluation methods with each other.

The presentations have indicated that some staff want to develop similar practices, and they are supported by mangers to meet on a monthly basis to undertake practice development plans. Practice development plans have included life story work, behavioral assessment, sensory techniques, communication strategies, structured day, and the introduction of Well- and Ill-Being (WIB) profiles.

Introduction of Positive Person Work

Many staff focus on the negative aspects of DCM evaluations. Discussion, challenges, and reflections often center on PDs. If staff believe that only the negative aspects of their care are under scrutiny, then they are in danger of feeling vulnerable to criticism. In the early days of DCM, the practice consequence of this focus on the negative produced staff action planning to address PDs while neglecting to develop the positive care aspects that were highlighted by evaluations. Although raising awareness of the effects of malignant social psychology is extremely important, it needs to be balanced by discussing the positive findings, particularly how such interactions are significant for people with dementia. During DCM evaluation feedback sessions, mappers now encourage debate regarding these issues and their relevance to person-centered care interventions and staff skills.

Kitwood (1997) began the exploration of *positive person work*. He described 12 types of positive interaction that have the potential to enhance people through "strengthening, positive feelings, nurturing ability or helping to heal psychological wounds" (p. 90). Ten types of positive interaction can be initiated by care staff, including validation, negotiation, holding, collaboration, play, timalation (directly engaging the senses), celebration, relaxation, recognition, and facilitation. These positive factors provide much detail and build on and develop staff practice (see Chapter 5). Kitwood illustrated these interactions within a vignette, which provided enough detail for an analysis of how these interactions are beneficial for people with dementia.

As of 2002, various ward teams within the Trust are implementing positive person work as part of appraisals and individual clinical supervision. The staff development opportunities of positive person work continue to develop. Many staff are unable to articulate dementia care specific skills. Nonetheless, it is evident in practice (especially during DCM evaluations) that many possess person-centered qualities and their skilled interventions with patients have therapeutic properties. Sustaining positive interactions with people who have dementia requires a great deal of commitment and skills from the care worker. The more severe the dementia, the greater the need for skilled therapeutic interactions.

The positive person work framework has enabled staff to reflect on and critically appraise their own practice in relation to their skills and to identify skills that they believe require development. Staff who need to develop specific therapeutic interventions can be linked to other staff who are able to demonstrate the specific skills. In addition, staff are encouraged to use a reflective journal to explore thoughts, experiences, and action plans. The journal can then be used as part of individual appraisal and supervision. The supervisor's role is to provide support and guidance in opportunities that focus on skills development.

Clinical Supervision for Mappers

Starting in 1996, DCM evaluations became an integral part of practice at the Trust. It became more evident that a number of professional practice and personal issues related to mapping had to be explored and resolved. It was decided that more time was needed to address these issues; therefore, the meeting times of the monthly DCM special interest group were extended. Through these discussions, it became clear that clinical supervision was the way to facilitate reflection, explore options, agree on resolutions, and offer mutual support.

As a group, the mappers reviewed the literature on clinical supervision and formulated a supervision contract that identified the purpose and format of the supervision (Hawkins & Shohet, 1989). The contract contained the following:

• The functions of the supervision, including professional issues, accountability issues related to roles, personal issues, and training and development issues

- Issues of attendance
- Confidentiality
- Roles and responsibilities of mappers

To provide a bit more insight to the contract, some of its components are described in detail next.

Professional Issues The focus of the professional function is advancing clinical and professional practice through critical exploration of roles and responsibilities and dilemmas in practice. This analysis is achieved through reflection and resolution in a number of areas. For example, one issue was informed consent (i.e., a patient's capacity to give consent to the mapping evaluations). After a discussion, it was agreed that mappers should introduce themselves and explain the purpose of the day to patients prior to and during mapping. Management staff are also encouraged to reinforce this information to care workers and patients prior to and during mapping. If an individual becomes distressed by being observed, then that observation will cease. If the individual continues to be distressed by mapping, then the DCM evaluation will stop.

Another example of a professional issue was the conflict between an individual's roles as a mapper and a staff member (e.g., nurse, occupational therapist). This conflict particularly related to intervention when mappers observed PDs and practice dilemmas during DCM evaluations. The resolution came through exploration of professional codes of conduct and responsibilities to ensure that residents are not harmed by poor care standards. A clearly defined procedure for dealing with unsafe practice and practice dilemmas during DCM evaluations was developed and included in the clinical supervision contract.

A third realm of professional function was the increased levels of activity in some clinical areas on the days of DCM evaluations. Resolution on this dilemma included mappers' supporting individual clinicians to sensitively address their issues of concern during DCM feedback presentations.

Personal Issues The focus of the personal function provides opportunities for mappers to explore feelings and emotions that result from their mapper role. One personal issue that has been addressed is the conflict between observing and participating in care delivery. Through reflection and critical discussion, the group considered the experiences of care staff. The focus of this resolution was to consider the purpose of mapping.

Another exploration involved relationships between mappers and residents and the mapping of one's clinical area. Critical exploration indicated that mappers who had in-depth knowledge of patients were using their knowledge and experience to influence WIB scores. Mappers also felt that mapping their own clinical area could lead to conflicts of interest. It was therefore agreed early on that mappers would not map their own clinical areas.

Training and Development Issues   The training and development function enables the continuous enhancements of skills and promotes evidence-based advanced practice. Some of these issues have included the interpretation and recording of a $+5$ level of well-being, the recording and feedback of PDs, and interactions with care staff during mapping and feedback. Role play and interrater reliability tests were utilized to address some of these issues.

Summary   Honest and open communication within supervision sessions has enabled the resolution of some sensitive and difficult issues. Certain issues raised during the supervision have been made the focus of further training and developmental programs for mappers and care staff. Formal evaluation of clinical supervision by mappers has been positive. Mappers have concluded that although many of the issues addressed are challenging, exploration and reflection have enabled personal and professional growth. Mappers are encouraged to keep reflective journals, which can be used to complement their professional development records.

Group Clinical Supervision

Following consultation with clinical staff, a framework was developed for the implementation of group clinical supervision for nursing staff. The framework's theoretical orientation was based on formative, restorative, and normative functions (Proctor, 1986).

Formative Function   The formative function focuses on how the supervised person works with residents. The function is related to the development of skills, understanding, and abilities. This is achieved through reflection and exploration of the supervised person's work in some of the following areas:

- Enhancing skills and evidence-based practice in person-centered assessment and interventions

- Identifying individualized resident needs within the assessment and demonstrating the relationship between assessment and person-centered interventions

- Developing critical thinking and problem-solving skills

Restorative Function   The restorative function facilitates reflection on and exploration of emotions that result from the nurse–resident relationship. Nurses working with people who have dementia are often affected by the residents' pain, distress, and disabilities. Therefore, emphasis was given to the following concepts:

- Addressing emotions and responses that are stimulated by the interaction with people who have dementia

- Developing coping strategies to deal with stress and anxiety that is related to working with people who have dementia

- Developing critical incident approaches within clinical practice. Within this framework, critical incidents are based on challenging resident–nurse communications. These are explored to develop an effective practical approach to ethically challenging communication issues.

- Establishing a working alliance with peers to provide opportunities for support, learning, and self-examination

Normative Function   The normative function provides a quality assurance system within the context of clinical supervision. Such supervision is achieved through

- Facilitating the critical examination of clinical decision making

- Exploring approaches to therapeutic clinical and person-centered interventions

- Enhancing the quality of life for older people with dementia

- Ensuring safe and effective clinical practice

Summary   In practice, group supervision usually occurs in a case presentation format. The format allows the opportunity to explore in detail person-centered assessment, interventions, and evaluation of care for the person with dementia. Individual care summaries from DCM evaluations are included to enhance this process. As of 2001, functional analysis/equivalence has been implemented as part of clinical supervision; such analysis attempts to address the functions served by challenging behavior (Stokes, 2001). The pursuit of explanations not only includes that which is observed but also explores the person-centered aspects of life history, abilities, needs, and so forth. This approach has enabled staff to explore and discuss creative person-centered explanations, which promote interventions that attempt to meet the needs of each individual with dementia.

Clinical Practice Developments

Changes in clinical practice include the development of an observer role during actual DCM evaluations. The observer's aim is to watch and make objective comments regarding care. This role allows the person to take a step back from direct care delivery and gain greater insight to the care being delivered.

The observer gives an alternative clinical perspective to supplement the DCM data. The observer, who is not a trained mapper, is nominated by the clinical team prior to the map. Support and guidance is offered prior and during the map by the managers and mappers. The person must be prepared to give feedback about the positive and negative observations and must have the ability to view care from the perspective of a person with dementia.

To assist in this process, observer guidelines have been formulated which provide a basis for feedback. Guidelines include observation on

- Positive events

- Interactions

- General activity/inactivity

- Environment

- Visitors

- Negative events

- General observations of individual patients and the group of patients

- General atmosphere of the clinical area

The clinical observer has become integral to the mapping process because he or she produces rich data and can give excellent feedback to the clinical team. Staff have also indicated that when a clinical observer is involved, they feel greater ownership of the DCM evaluation.

Another development in clinical practice is the formulation of action planning guidelines. These guidelines were developed following repeated requests from clinical staff to help them develop action plans following DCM evaluations. The guidelines encourage the teams to acknowledge and develop their strengths as well as their areas for improvement. The action plan provides the team with a clear focus for practice development.

CONCLUSION

It is important to acknowledge that DCM alone will not bring about all the changes needed to develop and sustain person-centered care practices within formal caregiving environments. Person-centered care involves a style of caring that emphasizes the therapeutic nurse–resident relationship. The relationship requires continuity of care and the acceptance of responsibility for the outcomes of care. This involves focusing on clinical effectiveness, patient outcomes, and evidence-based practice. Person-centered care is extremely demanding in terms of staff commitment, attitudes, and skills. Developments in person-centered care lead to further demands on staff as practice is continually challenged. It must be noted that not all staff members will be committed to working within a person-centered framework.

Developing person-centered care initiatives in practice requires a systematic approach, which includes staff development and practice development initiatives that are supported by the organization. This chapter has detailed a range of practice development and staff development initiatives that the Trust has utilized. The impact of these initiatives has led to cultural changes in staff's attitudes and knowledge. There is also a greater ownership of the person-centered philosophy, and creative practices are being implemented into care. DCM and person-centered care practices have raised staff's expectations in a range of different perspectives. As a result, continued organizational support is crucial to the ongoing development of person-centered care practices. Implementing such a strategy is costly in terms of time, commitment, and resources; however, the rewards are immense.

REFERENCES

Brooker, D., Forster, N., Banner, A., Payne, M., & Jackson, L. (1998). The efficacy of Dementia Care Mapping as an audit tool: Report of a 3 year British NHS Evaluation. *Ageing and Mental Health, 2*(1), 60–70.

Buckland, S. (1995). Dementia Care Mapping: Looking a bit deeper. *Signpost, 32,* 5–7.

Hawkins, P., & Shohet, R. (1989). *Supervision in the helping professions.* Buckingham, England: Open University Press.

Journal of Dementia Care. (1996–1997). *Person Centred Care Series.* London: Hawker Publications.

Killick, J. (1997). *You are words.* London: Hawker Publications.

Kitwood, T. (1997). *Dementia reconsidered: The person comes first.* Buckingham, England: Open University Press.

Loveday, B., & Kitwood, T. (1998). *Improving dementia care: A resource for training and personal development.* London: Hawker Publications.

Proctor, B. (1986). Supervision: A co-operative exercise in accountability. In M. Marken & M. Payne (Eds.), *Enabling and ensuring supervision in practice.* Leicester, England: National Youth Bureau, Council for Education and Training in Youth and Community Work.

Stokes, G. (2001). *Challenging behaviour in dementia: A person centred approach.* Bicester, England: Winslow Press.

Williams, J., & Rees, J. (1997). The use of Dementia Care Mapping as a method of evaluating care received by patients with dementia. *Journal of Advanced Nursing, 25,* 316–323.

III

POLICY AND
DEMENTIA CARE
MAPPING
PRINCIPLES

7

THE AUSTRALIAN
PERSPECTIVE ON
DEMENTIA CARE
MAPPING AND THE
LONG-TERM CARE FIELD

VIRGINIA MOORE

Dementia Care Mapping (DCM) is in its infancy in Australia. Dementia care, however, is like a normal, healthy teenager—struggling to find and assert its own identity and value among mature care services such as cancer care, cardiology, orthopedics, and pediatrics. Nonetheless, there are some excellent residential care facilities for people with dementia and some innovative and high-quality community-based services. Others require a lot of work to bring them up to a standard that supports the personhood of people with dementia. As of 2002, DCM use in Australia has been limited to residential facilities (group living facilities for older adults with high support needs). Therefore, this chapter only refers to the use of DCM with people with dementia living in residential care facilities, both high care (nursing facilities) and low care (hostels).

Like many other Western societies, Australia has yet to accept dementia without the accompanying fear, myths, and misunderstandings, which lead to its denial of dementia as a subject worthy of wholehearted support. The government, however, is well aware of the increasing number of older Australians and the potential impact of an aging society on future health care costs. Thus, Australia's federal government has significantly contributed to services for people with dementia since the early 1990s. In 1993, a national action plan for dementia was initiated, with the express goals of identifying key issues such as training needs, special design requirements, assessment, and ongoing management requirements. Some critical issues (in particular, training needs) were highlighted, and strategies to address these were implemented. The National Dementia Residential Training Initiative Evaluation Report (Commonwealth Department of Health and Ageing, 1998, March) collected anecdotal comments that indicated a moderate shift in staff attitudes and understanding. However, the report also recommended ongoing funding for staff training in this complex area. Although some significant progress has been made, it is still fair to say that the government has yet to articulate a long-term vision for the care of older adults with dementia in Australia.

To understand the potential for use of DCM within Australia's culture of care, a brief overview of the Australian system for long-term care (or "Aged Care") is necessary. The chapter begins with a summary outlining the framework within which services for people with dementia operate. It is within this arena that DCM operates as an evaluation tool and a change agent for care practices. Following this summary, some of the practical implications for the use of DCM are discussed within the context of organizational and systems culture.

STRUCTURE OF AUSTRALIA'S LONG-TERM CARE SYSTEM

On the one hand, residential care for older adults is the responsibility of Australia's federal government, which is based in Canberra. All legislative decisions and funding derive from this source. On the other hand, acute care and rehabilitation services come within the jurisdiction of the state governments. The majority of community support services are funded by the federal government but administered by the states under a commonwealth/state agreement. However, as an alternative to residential care, the federal government also funds and manages care packages that enable people to receive care in their own homes.

In 1987, radical changes occurred regarding how residential and community services were structured, funded, and audited. That system operated until 1997, when the Aged Care Act was passed and the current system came into operation. The following subsections summarize the current system.

Assessment and Referral

Initial assessment for dementia is generally made by the community medical practitioner. In some instances, referrals may come through the acute care system. For more detailed assessment, medical practitioners can refer to the Aged Care Assessment Teams (ACATs), which are based within regional health care areas. ACATs are comprised of geriatricians, registered nurses (RNs), social workers, and occupational therapists. Medical practitioners refer people to ACATs for assessment, recommendations, and referral to the service type required. All people seeking residential care must have an ACAT assessment and referral.

Community Care Services

Various types of community care services exist. Home and Community Care (HACC) services are funded to provide support for people in their own homes or within their own community (e.g., domiciliary nursing services, Meals on Wheels, day centers). Community Aged Care Packages (CACP) provide low care (hostel) level support to people in their own homes. This can range from shopping and meal preparation to personal care and medication supervision. Extended Aged Care at Home (EACH) packages provide high care (nursing facility) service to people within their own homes. This support includes supervision and care by an RN, plus support from care workers who provide the service under the RN's direction.

Residential Low Care and Residential High Care

Residential Low Care provides 24-hour supervision and support. Care is provided by care workers under supervision of a care coordinator. Professional support (e.g., from an RN or allied health professional) is provided on a request-for-service basis. Residential High Care provides 24-hour, 7-day per week care, within a group facility of up to 60 people, under the direct supervision of an RN, supported by registered allied health professionals, enrolled nurses, care workers, therapy assistants, and/or recreational ("diversional") therapy staff.

Medical Care

Medical care for people with dementia is provided by the medical practitioner of their choice. If specialist care is required, then the medical practitioner makes a referral to the appropriate specialist service.

Funding System

CACP, EACH, and residential services are funded separately but share one major feature. Funding is determined according to the assessed needs of each person using a specified system for assessment of need.

Community Care Services HACC is funded jointly by state and federal governments and administrated through the states. CACP and EACH are funded and administered by the federal government only. Both types of care packages are individually designed within a specified maximum number of hours per week.

Residential High Care and Residential Low Care Following admission to residential low or high care, each person's support needs are assessed over a 6-week period using a funding tool, the Resident Classification Scale (RCS; Commonwealth Department of Health and Ageing, 2001). Care needs are identified between Level 1 (*highest need*) and Level 8 (*lowest need*). Each level gives the care facility a specified amount of money per day for that person. In addition, a weekly fee is charged directly to each resident. The actual fee charged is determined by a means-tested assessment of the resident's financial assets.

Auditing Documentation of all residential care facilities is audited regularly to ensure that submitted RCS applications are accurate. Auditing is done at short notice and conducted on a random 10% of health records. Auditors have the authority to change the submitted level if documented evidence of the claims is not substantiated. Funding changes accordingly and is backdated if need be.

Accreditation Each residential facility must achieve accreditation to maintain eligibility for continued licensing and funding. Accreditation is based on a quality improvement approach and covers four standards and their accompanying subsections:

1. Management systems, staffing, and organizational development, with nine subsections

2. Health and personal care, with 17 subsections that cover all aspects of clinical care (including behavioral issues)

3. Resident lifestyle, with 10 subsections that cover aspects of lifestyle (including social and human needs areas)

4. Physical environments and safe systems, which encompass occupational safety and health, fire and security, infection control, and catering and linen services

Each standard also has three common subsections: continuous improvement, regulatory compliance, and education and staff development.

The accreditation process is exacting and can be achieved for 1- or 3-year periods. Accreditation details of each facility are available on the Internet for public access, allowing the public to make an informed preselection of facilities.

Services for People with Dementia Services for people with dementia are funded within the overall care framework for older adults. Individual providers make the choice to provide dementia-specific facilities or to provide an integrated model of care. This is done despite the fact that approximately 70% of all people in residential care settings have some form of dementia. Consequently, many facilities have integrated services. Others have areas designed specifically for people with dementia who are mobile and require a secure environment.

PRACTICAL CONSIDERATIONS FOR PROMOTING DEMENTIA CARE MAPPING

A number of factors influence the promotion of DCM in Australia, not the least of which is the country's geographical size. This, coupled with the relatively small and widely dispersed population, presents a challenge for equal service distribution. Australia is approximately 7,692,030 square kilometers in size (Australian Bureau of Statistics, 2001), roughly 75% of the size of the United States of America. In June 2000, Australia's population was 19.2 million (Australian Bureau of Statistics, 2001), compared with the U.S. population of approximately 281.4 million (U.S. Census Bureau, 2000).

Approximately 85% of the total Australian population lives within major cities, all of which (with the exception of Canberra) are on the coastal areas of the country. Rural communities range in size from major regional centers to small communities of 100–200 people. There is often considerable distance between centers, with people being far from the nearest services. All of these factors affect the way in which a method like DCM is introduced, implemented, and monitored in a care system.

In Australia, two areas have been using DCM since the late 1990s. On the east coast, Wylie (2000) used DCM in her doctoral thesis to measure the effectiveness of sensory enrichment programs on the well-being of people with dementia. This is the first research conducted in the Australian long-term care system that has used DCM to measure outcomes of client satisfaction. It is highly significant. The findings of this research are attracting considerable interest and, as a result, interest in person-centered care and DCM is growing.

Dr. Wylie continues to use person-centered care and DCM in her work as Nurse Educator at Allendale Aged Care Facility, in the Hunter Health Care region of New South Wales.

On the west coast, in Perth, the Brightwater Care Group facilities have used DCM to evaluate care. Brightwater has adopted the person-centered approach as its philosophy of care for all services. Brightwater Care Group is a large, not-for-profit organization with a history of long-term care for younger and older people with disabilities. Residential care, both high and low care, is provided for approximately 530 people living in 11 long-term care facilities throughout the Perth region. Services for a further 200 people are provided within their own homes. Approximately 60%–70% of these people have some form of dementia.

Until 2001, neither implementor of DCM had trainer status and there were no other trained users of DCM within Australia. Brightwater now has one qualified DCM trainer (me), with a second undertaking the training certificate, so it is possible to begin training care practitioners across the country. This will extend the use of DCM to quantify the quality of care. In turn, DCM is beginning to be used to determine directions for change and improvement based on feedback from the person with dementia and his or her experiences in the care setting.

This chapter's observations on how DCM fits within the Australia's long-term care system are based mainly on my experiences since 1999, when the tool was introduced at Brightwater. It was not until 2001 that DCM began to elicit wider interest in Australia.

CULTURAL CONSIDERATIONS FOR
PROMOTING DEMENTIA CARE MAPPING

This section discusses two cultural aspects that are pertinent to promoting DCM in Australia. First is the sensitivity of DCM to the emotional responses of people from different cultural backgrounds (i.e., individual cultural issues). Second is transferring an evaluation tool designed for one care system to another care system (i.e., care system cultural issues). Both aspects are detailed in the following subsections.

Individual Cultural Issues

Because DCM use in Australia is restricted to two registered mappers, the following comments can only be considered anecdotal and cannot be seen as more than preliminary observations. As one of the mappers, I have mapped people from Macedonian, Polish, English, Australian, Irish, and Italian backgrounds. In each instance, the Well- or Ill-Being (WIB) indicators listed in the DCM manual (Bradford Dementia Group, 1997) have provided a valuable reflection of the person's emotional status at the time of observation, contributing to effective care changes for the individual concerned. A number of people with dementia revert to using their first or native language, placing them at significant risk of social isolation within the residential setting due to language and/or cultural barriers. Although awareness of this issue is reasonably high, DCM has proved to be a useful tool in identifying specific issues for the individual that may easily be overlooked. If left unattended, this isolation can soon lead to withdrawal and apathy or, alternatively, can heighten the potential for anger and frustration, resulting in physical outbursts. The WIB indicators have provided valuable evidence of the person's response to his or her social environment and can therefore be used as a basis for care changes to promote well-being and reduce isolation.

Nevertheless, a note of caution is necessary. In Western societies at the beginning of the 21st century, the accepted model for aging promotes independence as a sign of wellness/well-being. Yet within some cultures, a "sickness/dependency" role is quite acceptable for older adults. In these cultures, people expect to be looked after and nurtured in their latter years and, thus, dependency is not feared (Trimboli, 2001). Thus, well-being indicators such as being helpful to others may be seen rarely, if at all. In these situations, the mapper must be extra vigilant to ensure that he or she maps the person's responses, not interpretations based on the mapper's cultural expectations. This area warrants further research.

As of 2002, DCM has not been carried out with members of Australia's indigenous community. Therefore, no data are available on this topic. Differences in nonverbal communication styles may well require more in-depth work before reliability of the method can be ensured for this group in Australia.

Care System Cultural Issues

A number of issues for promoting DCM result from the culture of the care system in Australia. Like some other countries, care facilities are owned by either not-for-profit organizations or private for-profit organizations. State governments own the few remaining government facilities, and most of these are in transition to private ownership. With funding tied to individual resident needs, there is a high risk of increased dependency levels being rewarded with increases in funding levels. Facilities must remain financially viable to continue operating, which puts pressure on staff to focus on maximum funding at the expense of optimum physical and emotional well-being.

Facilities must meet stringent standards in a number of areas. Many facilities provide both physical and social environments that positively support the well-being of people with dementia. The concept of measuring how the environment and the social psychology affect the person with dementia is perhaps less well understood. Some providers perceive that DCM is an expensive luxury that Australia's current system cannot afford. In many other instances, service providers are simply unaware that such a tool exists or how it can be used. There is, however, a growing awareness of and interest in the concept of using emotional responses as the measure of satisfaction from the consumer's point of view.

In addition, funding for residential services is so tightly monitored that service providers have difficulty replacing staff who leave for DCM's 3-day training course. Likewise, relieving staff from the floor to map for lengthy periods is another issue that must be negotiated carefully. The recommendation to conduct mapping for a minimum of 6 hours works against the acceptance of the tool. Releasing staff to map for this length of time is perceived as impractical and too costly in the current environment. Using DCM in a flexible, realistic, and responsive manner in relation to both funding and staffing issues is essential if use by direct care staff is to be achieved.

However, I believe that this goal can be achieved in the following ways:

- Use DCM to map specific times of the day that care staff find difficult. If the objective is clearly to identify issues that lead to direct solutions, then it is possible to negotiate for additional hours. This is particularly true when occupational health and safety issues are present.

- Negotiate between staff members to enable one member to be released to map residents with whom staff are experiencing particular problems.

- Target key times of the day (e.g., mealtimes) to identify possible improvements.

- Reach an agreement to rotate the mapping period through several different mappers to ensure that a longer period of time is observed.

Without this flexibility, it is doubtful that use of DCM by care staff in their own setting will be successful. Involvement with and support from research and development groups who may be able to provide mapping for longer periods will be essential for the successful introduction and ongoing use of the tool in Australia.

INCORPORATING DEMENTIA
CARE MAPPING INTO A CARE SYSTEM

For DCM to be successful within the Australian long-term care system (and perhaps in other countries seeking to implement DCM with limited resources and mappers) several key steps need to be achieved. These can be divided into two sections: the national level and the individual organizational level.

National Level

An ongoing partnership between east coast and west coast trainers must be established to ensure that consistency, reliability, and the integrity of the tool are maintained. This is already occurring, with both parties committed to the concept. Links with universities must also be established to further research and develop DCM in the Australian long-term care environment. Initial links have begun, following the interest expressed by several universities on the east and west coasts. In addition, an implementation plan and timetable need to be developed, including conference presentations, workshops, and clinical training sessions with interested professional groups. Finally, establishing a national DCM strategic development group incorporating the key areas of clinical, research, and community support groups is essential to ensure that DCM users stay abreast of changes and development. As the peak body representing people with dementia and their care workers, the Alzheimer's Association would be the preferred community representative.

Individual Organizational Level

DCM must be actively promoted in conjunction with the person-centered approach to care. The person-centered philosophy is consistent with the requirements of accreditation standards and provides an excellent framework for care practice rationale. It clearly outlines the consequence for the person with dementia if personhood is ignored. These consequences are measurable in financial and human cost.

In addition, it is necessary to clearly define how DCM can help direct positive changes and add value to life for the person with dementia and to the staff working with him or her. This needs to be done in a variety of ways, both formal and informal. The evidence that DCM produces should also be directly connected to the Australian Accreditation process. The data collected and the subsequent care plan and care practice changes are consistent with the continuous improvement model required for Australian Accreditation (see Chapter 5 for discussion of how this can be achieved). DCM provides the evidence required to substantiate the continuous improvement clause of Standard 3: Resident Lifestyle (Commonwealth Department of Health and Ageing, n.d.).

For DCM to be successful within any organization, support from senior management is essential before it is introduced. DCM is a powerful tool that, unless introduced in a structured and planned way, can leave care workers frustrated and disillusioned. It is essential that management has a full understanding of the process and the support mechanisms that need to be in place before investing in staff training. This type of support is critical for DCM to be effective in the long term.

Finally, the cost of training has to be made affordable within the existing, extremely tight financial structure. Service providers have to be realistic in prioritizing funds. Training costs sit alongside a number of other priorities. Providers must be clearly convinced that their investment will pay off, in terms of both resident well-being and a balanced budget. This is simply responsible management.

A number of points presented in this subsection are consistent with those presented by Kitwood (1997). If management lacks a genuine understanding of the true implications of DCM, then it is doubtful that any lasting change will occur. The risk is that staff will try their hardest to create the change and then become disillusioned if this is not achieved. In turn, DCM may become the scapegoat for staff frustrations and management's perception that it is "just another tool." A carefully planned and systematic approach is required for DCM to become securely embedded into an organization's culture. This process needs to closely involve all of the relevant groups within the organization, from clinical managers to human resources and finance personnel, as DCM has implications for all of these areas.

PRACTICAL EXAMPLE OF THE APPLICATION PROCESS

The Brightwater Care Group in Western Australia has demonstrated how DCM can be implemented. A planned approach was drawn up. DCM sits within this process as the means of measuring the changes and promoting further change in care practices. It was agreed that this approach would be implemented across a 2- to 3-year period and that it had to fit with other developments within the organization. All points, which are detailed in the following discussion, were either completed or are in progress as of 2002.

One element of the plan was an audit of existing services to identify the gaps in services, with recommendations for improvement. Among these recommendations: Identify a philosophy of care for dementia services and further explore the DCM process.

All executive and senior managers agreed to adopt the person-centered approach as the organization's philosophy. In turn, a three-tiered training approach was created as part of the annual training budget for use in all of the long-term care facilities. Level 1 of training is a 12-hour basic training program based on person-centered care for people with dementia. This program is attended by all staff. At Level 2, key people are selected to be trained in DCM and later take lead roles with staff. The dementia services consultant supports these staff. Level 3 involves 6-hour workshops for all senior managers, learning and development co-coordinators, and senior clinical staff to discuss the implications of adopting the person-centered approach. Workshops address management issues, including the staff support levels needed for implementing this approach. A plan for addressing these issues is then drawn up. These workshops are to be held at least annually to review progress.

To ensure widespread understanding, relative and resident meetings at each site were to include explanatory sessions. To ensure the plan's ability to provide high-quality person-centered care to people with dementia, an introductory session on the person-centered approach was also made part of the regular orientation program for all new staff. In addition, dementia-specific competency assessment was introduced for care staff.

Another component of the approach was a "site key person" system. This concept was initiated to ensure that resource people were trained and available as the first point of contact for each site. The site key person system has since been used successfully for areas requiring clinical expertise, such as continence and infection control.

Furthermore, a dementia steering group was launched, with representation from all sections and levels of the organization (including the At Home Services sector). This group was to be responsible for drawing up policies and procedures specific to dementia care practices and overseeing their implementation.

Finally, an agreement was made regarding research. Brightwater decided to actively seek research partners within the academic environment to collect data. This data, in turn, could be used to supplement data collected by the care staff.

CONCLUSION

DCM reflects and evaluates care against the philosophy of a person-centered approach (Kitwood, 1997). It cannot operate in isolation from this approach. Both person-centered care and DCM (as an evaluation and a change-agent tool) are consistent with and fit closely with Australia's system for accrediting long-term care programs. DCM provides quantifiable evidence of improvements in care practices based on the responses shown by people with dementia. It fits well within the overall system culture of long-term care for older adults.

For DCM to be successfully introduced and accepted within a wide circle of service providers, however, it needs to prove itself to be cost-effective and achievable within the existing staffing constraints. Both proprietors and staff must be convinced that DCM will provide valuable data that can be used effectively to create achievable changes within the existing system, which is currently under enormous pressure.

The key to this is proving that DCM can be used flexibly within the care environment to create staff awareness of how the social environment affects residents. Within residential facilities, systematically observing and collecting data for short periods of time (e.g., 30 minutes) can significantly raise staff awareness. These observation times can target recognized "problem" periods over the course of the day to identify the real issues relating to that time or situation. The information gained can be used to plan changes in response to specifically identified problems. If supported by management, then longer periods of mapping can be conducted and staff time can be covered to enable this.

With the use of DCM in its infancy, it is possible to introduce it systematically as a valuable adjunct to the accreditation process and as a change-agent tool for care practices. Developing key links with universities and other research facilities to continue developing the tool within the Australian environment is essential to provide reliable data. In turn, this data can be used to influence substantial change at a government policy level to effect long-term and permanent improvement for people with dementia who live in Australia.

REFERENCES

Australian Bureau of Statistics. (2001). *ABS statistics*. Retrieved April 4, 2002, from http://www.abs.gov.au/

Bradford Dementia Group. (1997). *Evaluating dementia care: The DCM method* (7th ed.). Bradford, England: University of Bradford.

Commonwealth Department of Health and Ageing, Aged and Community Care Division. (n.d.). *Aged Care Act 1997: Principles*. Retrieved October 21, 2001, from http://www.health.gov.au:80/acc/legislat/aca1997/prindex.htm

Commonwealth Department of Health and Ageing, Aged and Community Care Division. (1998, March). Impact of the NRDTI dementia care training on work practices (Chapter 4). In *The evaluation of the National Dementia Residential Training Initiative report.* Retrieved October 2001, from http://www.health.gov.au:80/acc/reports/nrdti/contents/chap4.htm

Commonwealth Department of Health and Ageing, Aged and Community Care Division. (1998, April). Contents. In *Extended aged care at home packages: Pilot guidelines for service providers.* Retrieved October 22, 2001, from http://www.health.gov.au:80/acc/guidelns/eachp/eachguid.htm

Commonwealth Department of Health and Ageing, Aged and Community Care Division. (1999, May). *Community care packages: Program guidelines.* Retrieved October 21, 2001, from http://www.health.gov.au:80/acc/commcare/cacp/guide1.htm

Commonwealth Department of Health and Ageing, Aged and Community Care Division. (1999, December). *Glossary for residential care manual.* Retrieved October 21, 2001, from http://www.health.gov.au:80/acc/manuals/rcm/contents/glossary.htm

Commonwealth Department of Health and Ageing, Aged and Community Care Division. (1999, December). *Residential care manual* (Rev. ed.). Retrieved October 22, 2001, from http://www.health.gov.au/acc/publicat/sppubs.htm

Commonwealth Department of Health and Ageing, Aged and Community Care Division. (2001, December). Classification Appraisal. In *Residential Care Manual.* Retrieved April 10, 2002, from http://www.health.gov.au/acc/manuals/rcm/rcmindx1.htm

Kitwood, T. (1997). *Dementia reconsidered. The person comes first.* Buckingham, England: Open University Press.

Trimboli, C. (2001). *How well are occupational therapists meeting the needs of their culturally diverse population?* "A Banquet of Mental Health" Conference, Bunbury, Western Australia.

U.S. Census Bureau. (2000). *United States Census 2000.* Retrieved April 4, 2002, from http://www.census.gov/main/www/cen2000.html

Wylie, K. (2000). *Valuing sensation and sentience in dementia care.* Unpublished doctoral thesis, University of Newcastle, New South Wales, Australia.

8

GOVERNMENT POLICY AND MEDICAL TRADITIONS IN HONG KONG

CORDELIA MAN-YUK KWOK

The positive experience of applying Dementia Care Mapping (DCM) in Hong Kong since 1999, as shown by its compatibility with traditional medical models of care in local settings, is discussed in this chapter. Included in the discussion are the strengths and limitations of the method in the Chinese context. The chapter also explores the application of the method within Chinese medical traditions and the main challenges of integrating DCM into Chinese society.

DEMENTIA IN HONG KONG

The development of dementia services in Hong Kong Special Administrative Region (HKSAR) began with the changeover of sovereignty in 1997. HKSAR was under British rule for more than 100 years before it was returned to Chinese sovereignty in 1997. Therefore, to a certain extent, an international system and model of health and social service has influenced Hong Kong.

HKSAR has a population of 6.7 million and is rapidly aging. Ninety-six percent of its population is ethnic Chinese (Census and Statistics Department,

2001). The number of people older than 65 years has increased to 11% of the total population. The prevalence of moderate to severe dementia in Hong Kong is 6% for those age 70 or older; it is estimated to be 4% for those age 65. About 45% of the individuals with dementia live in residential care homes (Chiu et al., 1998). A community survey found that 25% of adults age 60 and older have some degree of cognitive impairment, and 5% of those have moderate or severe cognitive impairment (Hong Kong Council of Social Service, 1997). In 1998, another survey conducted in 25 day care centers for older adults revealed that 22.6% had cognitive impairments (Working Group on Dementia, 1999).

HONG KONG SPECIAL ADMINISTRATIVE REGION GOVERNMENT POLICY ON DEMENTIA CARE

As in other developed countries, changes in demographics and technologies and rising costs make dementia care one of the main challenges for care workers, clinicians, practitioners, researchers, managers, and policy makers in Hong Kong (see Chapter 9). Until 1997, however, service development in dementia care was neglected in Hong Kong. The Elderly Commission was established in 1997 to focus on policy and lead strategic directions for elderly services. Medical services, community support services, legal issues, and new initiatives are being established or are in progress to address the inadequate quantity and quality of existing services (Chiu & Zhang, 2000).

In Hong Kong, caring for older people is considered a fundamental feature of a compassionate and caring society. The government policy of HKSAR aims to be responsive to the changing needs of the growing number of older adults and provides appropriate, innovative, cost-effective services to those with care needs. Dementia care in Hong Kong, however, has had a late start compared with the Western world. Since 1998, remarkable progress has been made toward new initiatives to support older adults (see Table 8.1). In particular, since 1999, DCM and the experiences of using it in Hong Kong have been disseminated at conferences and local seminars.

The Working Group on Dementia was set up under the Elderly Commission in August 1998. Members of the Working Group include members of the Elderly Commission, medical and social work professionals, academics, and representatives of relevant government departments. The Working Group aims to identify the care needs of people with dementia and the support services that their care workers require and to make recommendations on the provision of relevant services (Working Group on Dementia, 1999). Professional advocacy, especially by psychogeriatricians, has greatly influenced the devel-

Table 8.1. Significant dementia care developments in the Hong Kong Special Administrative Region

1993	Hong Kong Hospital Authority established psychogeriatric teams to serve different regions and provide services to patients with dementia and functional psychiatric illness. Included were inpatient, outpatient, consultation, and limited day hospital services, as well as outreach programs to assess and treat individuals living in residential facilities.
	The first memory clinics for early diagnosis of and intervention for dementia were established.
1994	Hong Kong Alzheimer's Disease and Brain Failure Association was established.
1998	The first Psychogeriatric Day Care Centre and Resources Centre for Dementia were set up to care for residents with psychological and behavior problems and to support family caregivers.
1999	The government provided the Dementia Supplement, which enables the service providers to employ additional staff—such as occupational therapists, social workers, and nurses—to provide better care and training for the residents with dementia.
	The University of Hong Kong Department of Social Work and Social Administration set up the Centre on Ageing to promote and develop geronotological research, education, services, and aging policy to enhance the physiological, psychological, and social well-being of older adults.
	A media source, Announcement of Public Interests (APIs), began promoting activities about and exhibitions on dementia, including information on the detection of dementia and care for people who have it.
	Eighteen Elderly Health Centres and 18 Visiting Health Teams were formed to provide multidisciplinary primary health care services to older adults. Services included the identification of risk factors for vascular dementia and the early detection of cognitive impairments through health screenings. Appropriate assessment, health education support groups, and wellness programs were provided for older individuals and their family members. Specialist referrals were provided, if necessary, for further evaluation and care.
	Support centers were set up to provide counseling to family caregivers, organize support groups, and offer training sessions on practical skills in caring for people with dementia.
	A 3-year pilot project was formed to set up dementia-specific units in day care centers and residential care homes. The goal of the project was to provide care services especially for people with dementia by offering tailor-made training and specialized programs and facilities (e.g., reality orientation, sensory stimulation, wandering paths, orientation signs in corridors and rooms). In 2002, a consultancy study will evaluate the effectiveness of these pilot projects and give recommendations for their long-term operation.
2000	The Department of Psychiatry at the Chinese University of Hong Kong established a dementia center to provide day care/respite services, staff training for care workers, and education and research programs.

opment of dementia services and government policy decisions. The Elderly Commission identified as priorities for future work the long-term care for older adults with special needs (e.g., dementia care), the financing of care, and quality assurance in residential care homes. Quality of life (QOL) is the central theme of the organization's work (Elderly Commission, 2001).

DEMENTIA CARE MAPPING'S COMPATIBILITY
WITH TRADITIONAL MEDICAL MODELS OF CARE

Dementia care programs and the use of DCM are in their infancy in Hong Kong. However, the most exciting and valuable contribution from using DCM is the promotion of QOL for people with dementia. This is achieved by enhancing meaningful activities and positive behaviors. Increased emphasis is placed on personhood and daily competencies (Kwok, 2001a, 2001b), as well as on intervention for behavioral and psychological symptoms of dementia (BPSD). BPSD present the greatest challenges in caring for people with dementia in local clinical settings (Lam, Tang, Leung, & Chiu, 2001) and dramatically affect the QOL of both patients and care workers.

Medical services have been the primary channel for introducing DCM in Hong Kong. DCM has been applied in three different facilities in the public sector: 1) psychogeriatric day care centers for people with dementia, 2) pilot projects of specific dementia units in day care centers, and 3) residential care homes. The objective is to evaluate the quality of the care in the facilities that voluntarily participated (Lee, 2001). Care workers in the public sector receive training in caring for people with dementia. The DCM data suggest that two facilities are good and one day center is excellent. However, the results may not be representative of care provision across Hong Kong because these are Hong Kong's model facilities.

Quality dementia care is a fundamental aspect of medical services. DCM has been applied in dementia units as a formal method to assess quality of care (Kwok, 2000). This has led to the identification of potential mechanisms for improving staff responses to challenging behaviors, including the promotion of positive behaviors and clinical supervision of staff (see Chapters 4 and 6). It is easy for mappers to highlight inadequate care provision, but it is not easy to make changes and DCM often fails to provide staff with alternative strategies.

In the facilities using DCM in Hong Kong, care routines were rearranged to follow the interest and pace of each individual with dementia. Both group and individual Well- or Ill-Being (WIB) values increased over successive DCM cycles. Time spent on well-being promotion activities increased without additional staff time and resources (Kwok, 2001b). Therefore, the data do not suggest the need for additional funding to improve services. Rather, service providers need to find new ways of working. DCM is unique and addresses the intricacy of evaluation, especially in how people who have dementia cope with it through the dynamic interaction among activities, participation, and the environment.

Carr and colleagues (2001) regarded the individual construct as essential for QOL measurement. The DCM process requires the mapper to put him- or herself into the place of the person with dementia and to consider care within that person's frame of reference. This is important for QOL measurement, as it enables an understanding of the experiences of people with dementia. As a result, the underlying reasons for a behavior can be investigated and addressed—a crucial aspect of dementia care.

Mapping Challenging Behavior

The International Psychogeriatric Association coined the phrase *behavioral and psychological symptoms of dementia (BPSD)* to describe challenging behavior in people with dementia (Finkel, Costa de Silva, Cohen, Miller, & Sartorius, 1996). BPSD include agitation, aggression, delusions, hallucinations, depression, apathy, sleep disturbances, and sexually inappropriate behaviors. BPSD are common, and their burden on people with dementia and care workers is well documented. These difficulties occur in up to 90% of people with dementia (Herrmann & Black, 2000). The behaviors are the most common reason for psychiatric referral, treatment with psychotropic drugs, and institutionalization (Steele, Rouner, Chase, & Folstein, 1990).

Lam and colleagues (2001) examined the BPSD profile for Chinese patients in a psychogeriatric unit in Hong Kong. They found that 61% had aggressive behavior, 32% had delusions, 15% had hallucinations, 54% had activity disturbances, 44% had sleep disturbances, 24% had affective disturbances, and 19% had anxiety and phobias. The study also revealed that up to 67.5% of patients with BPSD live in residential facilities.

A full and careful assessment of possible physical, psychological, and environmental factors is essential, as BPSD may have complex etiologies (Ballard, O'Brien, James, & Swann, 2001). However, clinicians should not view behavioral symptoms in isolation; rather, challenging behaviors should be understood in the context of the person's life. Numerous measures are used to describe and monitor behavioral symptoms. However, most are specifically designed to measure the manifestations of dementia; few are used to examine the impact of environment and psychosocial factors on people with dementia. Neglecting analysis of the detrimental effect of negative psychosocial or environmental factors may distort the therapeutic effect of treatments. More than any other instrument, using DCM has improved the ability to detect such external factors on individual well-being.

DCM is also compatible with the systematic "4D" approach, which professionals in Hong Kong use in their clinical practice to 1) define and describe, 2) decode, 3) devise a treatment plan, and 4) determine whether the treatment works (Rabins, Lyketsos, & Steele, 1999). The information derived from the medical condition, medication, cognitive disorder, psychiatric syndrome, and DCM map provides data on the environment and care worker approach. This is helpful for comprehensively decoding the causes of challenging behaviors and devising a treatment plan.

Environmental factors are analyzed by observing Personal Detractions (PDs) and by noting WIB categories that suggest that an individual's personhood has not been sustained, such as C (Cool—being socially uninvolved and withdrawn), D (Distress—expressing unattended stress), U (Unresponded to—communicating without receiving a response), and W (Withstanding—engaging repetitive self-stimulation). DCM "sharpens our eyes" and gives a chance to solve problems, provide timely intervention, or seek expert input. Moreover, the direct observation of behavior of people of dementia is often the only means to evaluate the impact of therapeutic intervention (Perrin, 1998).

The strategies of the Hong Kong government and Hospital Authority are "aging in place" and creating seamless health care by 1) restructuring and reorganizing medical services in collaboration with other providers and care workers in the community and 2) involving community members in the health care decision-making and delivery process (Hong Kong Hospital Authority, 2000). As of 2002, outreach services to Hong Kong's residential facilities is the major component of psychogeriatric services, with a strong educational element in the understanding and management of challenging behavior. Along those lines, DCM has been conducted in facilities and has given meaningful input to training and education programs. The mapping results provided information for staff to analyze their approaches and the responses of the individuals, as well as how to modify and fine-tune program schedules (Kwok, 2002; Lee, 2001).

Facilitating Individualized Programs Individualized programs offer the greatest prospect for therapeutic success (Burns, 1999). They provide an appropriate, flexible, and personalized approach. This is important for providing a tailored care package and monitoring the effectiveness of nonpharmacological interventions, especially regarding environmental modifications such as changing staff approaches (Ballard, O'Brien, James, & Swann, 2001).

A WIB score reflects a person's response to all interventions, including pharmacological interventions. In Hong Kong, using the language of WIB values and Behavior Category Codes (BCC) enables focused intervention for individuals (see Chapter 5). It also helps to reduce detrimental effects from the environment through observation and analysis of care worker behavior. In addition, it identifies and suggests strategies to prevent resident aggression and catastrophic reactions (Kwok, 2001a).

Providing Care Worker Training in Behavior Management Skills
Since the late 1990s, most interventions have focused on modifying the role of

care workers as "interventionists" of challenging behaviors and on the growing awareness of how their interactions with residents can act as antecedents and consequences, thereby strongly influencing the occurrence of behavior problems (Burgio & Fisher, 2000). Furthermore, positive behavior interactions between nursing home staff and residents were associated with a high degree of perceived staff involvement in decision-making processes, responsibility, and support (Cole, Scott, & Skelton-Robinson, 2000). In Hong Kong, most of the staff working in the residential facilities do not have training and experience in psychiatry. However, conventional education alone appears to be of limited value, as it has little impact on care worker well-being or behavioral symptoms of people with dementia (Coen et al., 1999). The intervention programs that have reported positive results are mostly comprehensive and multidimensional.

The data collected by DCM are concrete and allow feedback. Discussions of observations enable the support and development of skills from newly acquired knowledge and core information. DCM highlights the key features for change and development in care practice, and such possibilities do not exist in other programs and systems.

The DCM procedure is a developmental process (see Table 3 in the Introduction) and is well-matched with the commonly used contemporary management approach, the Just-In-Time (JIT) philosophy. The JIT approach involves eliminating unnecessary items and enriching specific goals, including the involvement of staff in the operation and the drive for continuous improvement (Cheng & Podolsky, 1996). In clinical practice in Hong Kong, frontline colleagues in some facilities are empowered with essential information (including the clinical findings to support it) to make appropriate interventions. They also consider enhanced resident enjoyment a sign of positive intervention outcome. The well-being that they observe from the responses and experiences of people with dementia is the best evidence supporting the endeavors of these frontline "interventionists."

Promoting Positive Behavior

In the care of people with dementia, positive behaviors are frequently ignored and challenging behaviors are the foci for interventions. As care responds to behavior problems, the essential goals of care—such as enhancing QOL and maximal functional independence—can be lost. Instead of asking, "How can we cope with negative or challenging behavior?" Sifton raised the more important question: "How can we support positive behavior engagement in meaningful activities?" (2000, p. 12). Using DCM to support positive behaviors may be one answer. DCM observations highlight many resident possibilities and strengths that were previously neglected. It provides new opportunities and spaces for true individualized programs and dementia services development. Moreover, creativity is an indispensable element of motivation and something that most people enjoy. Using DCM in Hong Kong has improved QOL for residents and has empowered caregiving professionals.

Reducing Excess Dependency and Promoting Everyday Competence

Functional decline is a significant indicator of dementia. The main factors contributing to excess disability are untreated medical and psychiatric conditions such as depression and ineffective caregiving strategies in activities of daily living (ADL; Larson, 1997). Thus, in Hong Kong, rehabilitation and caregiving strategies for people with dementia are focusing on maximizing abilities, daily competence, and life skills. Increased independence in ADL can be achieved without increasing disruptive behaviors, and it can foster appropriate requests for task-related help during caregiving (Rogers et al., 2000). DCM addresses this aspect through PDs, such as disempowerment, outpacing, and disparagement. Recording PDs highlights caregiving practices characterized by "not allowing a person to use the abilities that they do have; failing to help them to complete actions that they have initiated . . . [or doing so] at a rate too fast for a person to understand; putting them under pressure" and giving messages of incompetence and uselessness (Bradford Dementia Group, 1997, p. 57).

Furthermore, everyday competence is a transactional perspective of a person and his or her environment; it involves the active adaptation to a variety of environmental conditions (Diehl, 1998). Diehl advocated everyday competence as the future direction of health services for older adults. It motivates individuals to fully utilize their potential or capability to perform certain tasks. In turn, this action involves a person's physical, psychological (i.e., cognitive and emotional), and social functioning and influences the individual's day-to-day behavior. DCM fits with this concept because it examines the conditions and consequences of everyday behavior at different perspectives and levels with BCC and WIB values. In addition, DCM's underlying philosophy places much emphasis on holistic care and maintaining a balanced range of activities.

CONSIDERATIONS WHEN USING DEMENTIA CARE MAPPING IN MEDICAL SETTINGS

In Hong Kong, there are clinical protocols, guidelines, and audits to facilitate the quality of practice and to assist decision making. Physical and mental status assessments, neuropsychological testing, and other investigations form this groundwork and are extremely important to support the analysis of the behaviors and needs of people with dementia. DCM is one of the methods used to supplement the missing link between the bureaucrats and the caregiving process.

The DCM data should be carefully interpreted along with other details about individuals, including their physical and psychological conditions, when the method is used in clinical settings. For example, taking psychotropic drugs has been shown to significantly reduce well-being, increase time of withdrawn behavior, and reduce the proportion of time spent actively or passively engaged in activities; it places people particularly at risk for ill-being (Ballard, O'Brien, James, Mynt, et al., 2001). Therefore, signs of ill-being, such as being socially uninvolved or sleeping for long periods of the day, may not relate to the direct care approach in some situations.

One limitation is that DCM only assesses what occurs in communal areas. The observation of private areas, such as bathrooms, constitutes an abuse of the DCM method. Yet, aggression may often be noted during physical activities (e.g., bathing, dressing) that take place in private areas. This limits the application of DCM in behavior assessment.

Feedback sessions should be highly educational and professional to promote the application concepts, knowledge, and evidence to practice situations, especially regarding individualized care/goal planning on behavioral intervention. The evaluators need to mediate feedback sessions. In Hong Kong, senior staff or nurse specialists generally serve as the mappers. These people typically influence professional development as well.

Doody and colleagues recommended graded assistance as a strategy for dementia care. It can be "assistance from verbal prompts to physical demonstration, physical guidance, partial physical demonstration, partial physical assistance, and complete physical assistance aimed to provide the least amount of help possible" (2001, p. 1163). Graded assistance should be used to increase functional independence as guidelines. These strategies have been developing as positive events coding categories to enhance care practice in Hong Kong.

CHALLENGES OF INTEGRATING DEMENTIA CARE MAPPING IN CHINESE SOCIETY

Despite the advantages of using DCM in Hong Kong, Chinese society presents certain challenges for implementing the method. Further research is definitely needed to establish whether DCM is valid across ethnic and cultural groups. The following subsections discuss these issues of language, culture, and a non-Western concept of well-being.

Language

As of 2002, mappers in Hong Kong do not go through the whole framework of DCM to become approved trainers. Even if they did, most materials on DCM are in English, and English is not the primary language in China. The availability of Chinese articles on DCM is very limited. This has affected the development and dissemination of DCM in Hong Kong. In the meantime, only BCC, WIB, and PD codes have been translated for the purposes of communicating with others about DCM's philosophies and sharing data. Difficulties have been experienced in translating coding, terminology, and concepts. There is no similar system in the Chinese language, which could complement the use of alphabetic memory cues for BCC coding. Mappers and colleagues are encouraged to learn the BCC coding in English and to supplement coding descriptions with Chinese explanations. This bilingual approach is the best possible solution.

Culture

In Hong Kong, disempowerment, outpacing, and infantilization are the most commonly observed PDs, and most of them are done unintentionally. Other forms of PDs are rarely noted. Most professionals, including mappers, are uncomfortable with openly "digging up" PDs. In Chinese society, criticism is considered aggressive, and most Chinese individuals are concerned with maintaining peace and harmony. Perhaps in Chinese society, it would be more constructive to map the positive behavior of staff to recognize their efforts and support their appropriate practices.

In addition, there are several hundred identifiable minority groups in mainland China. Strictly speaking, the Chinese people are not a homogenous group. However, many people "feel they are Chinese because they share traditional roots, Confucian thought, or a cultural heritage of three thousand years" (Lin, Tseng, & Yen, 1995, p. 9). Thus, Chinese culture is unique. Furthermore, cultural differences arise when using instruments that were developed in other countries, especially in using observation to measure subjective qualities such as QOL or well-being. Communication patterns, social interactions, and expressions of feelings and moods are more implicit among the Chinese. Chow (1987) pointed out that countries cannot simply follow other countries' policies on population aging but that each must be aware of its own special traditions and culture; what is inherited from the past exerts an influence on the ways that older adults currently are treated in society. Therefore, using DCM to measure the experience of Chinese people with dementia and the interactions among environments offers uncertain validity.

Non-Western Concept of Well-Being

Evidence of well-being is the essence of DCM, but its appropriateness for Chinese society has been questioned. These doubts especially center on some indicators of well-being, such as assertiveness and "being able to express wishes, humor, creative self-expression, initiating social contact, affection, [and] expressing a full range of emotions, both positive and negative" (Bradford Dementia Group, 1997, p. 5). In contrast to Western societies, the Chinese tend to be emotionally reserved, introverted, fond of tranquility, overly considerate, socially overcautious, and self-restrained (Song, 1985, cited in Tseng & Wu, 1985). As a result, DCM cannot be automatically generalized to Chinese society.

The DCM participants' scores on the Cantonese Version of Mini-Mental Status Examination (CMMSE; Chiu, Lee, Chung, & Kwong, 1994) ranged from 6 to 16. These scores indicated a moderate to severe degree of dementia. The participants' interaction patterns and responses were direct and explicit and sometimes appeared "assertive" instead of "accommodative," which does not seem to be the cultural context for older Chinese adults. Are the data related to the residents' impaired higher functioning skills? Are cultural influences not as important when applied to people with dementia? It is important to address all of these questions.

CONCLUSION

DCM does not challenge the traditional medical model in Hong Kong; in fact, it enriches and complements dementia care services. In Hong Kong, DCM is not simply used to evaluate quality care. By maximizing capability in daily living, it has also contributed to the promotion of activities that enhance well-being. DCM observations have been used as an assessment instrument for describing the behavior of people with dementia, as well as to monitor and document the effect of the behavioral interventions and to support training on behavioral issues.

It is important to interpret DCM data along with other information about individuals. In addition, high educational and professional elements are needed in training to enhance service changes. DCM is probably the most useful method for doing so within the clinical setting (Brooker, 1995). Yet, challenges do exist regarding language, culture, and China's non-Western concept of well-being. As a result, DCM's validity in Chinese society is uncertain, and further research is definitely needed to establish whether DCM is valid across ethnic and cultural groups.

As dementia care services and DCM are developing in Hong Kong, certain areas require further study to support the application of DCM in a traditional medical setting and to facilitate its fit with HKSAR's governmental policy. More data are needed to describe the impact of DCM on improved interventions for challenging behavior, especially in reducing the use of antipsychotic medications and physical restraints, effectiveness on care worker training in behavioral intervention, and improvements in services and QOL.

REFERENCES

Ballard, C., O'Brien, J., James, I., Mynt, P., Lana, M., Potkins, D., Reichelt, K., Lee, L., Swann, A., & Fossey, J. (2001). Quality of life for people with dementia living in residential and nursing home care: The impact of performance on activities of daily living, behavioral and psychological symptoms, language skills, and psychotropic drugs. *International Psychogeriatrics, 13*(1), 93–106.

Ballard, C., O'Brien, J., James, I., & Swann, A. (2001). *Dementia: Management of behavioural and psychological symptoms.* New York: Oxford University Press.

Bradford Dementia Group. (1997). *Evaluating dementia care: The DCM method* (7th ed.). Bradford, England: University of Bradford.

Brooker, D. (1995). Looking at them, looking at me: A review of observational studies into the quality of institutional care for elderly with dementia. *Journal of Mental Health, 4,* 145–156.

Burgio, L.D., & Fisher, S. (2000). Application of psychosocial interventions for treating behavioral and psychological symptoms of dementia. *International Psychogeriatrics, 12*(Suppl. 1), 351–358.

Burns, A. (1999). Non-pharmacological treatment of BPSD in dementia. Report on behavioural and psychological symptoms of dementia (BPSD): A clinical and research update. *International Psychogeriatrics, 11*(Suppl. 1), 88.

Carr, A., Gibson, B., & Robinson, P. (2001). Is quality of life determined by expectations or experience? *British Medical Journal, 322,* 1240–1243.

Census and Statistics Department, Hong Kong Special Administrative Region. (2001, October 26). *Summary results of 2001 population census.* Retrieved April 3, 2002, from http://www.info.gov.hk/censtatd/eng/press/population/01c/press261001_index.html

Cheng, T.C.E., & Podolsky, S. (1996). *Just-in-time manufacturing: An introduction* (2nd ed.). San Diego: Chapman & Hall.

Chiu, H.F.K., Lam, L.C.W., Chi, I., Leung, T., Li, S.W., Law, W.T., Chung, D.W.S., Fung, H.H.L., Kan, P.S., Lum, C.M., Ng, J., & Lau, J. (1998). Prevalence of dementia in Chinese elderly in Hong Kong. *Neurology, 50,* 1002–1009.

Chiu, H.F.K., Lee H.C., Chung, W.S., & Kwong, P.K. (1994). Reliability and validity of the Cantonese version of the Mini-Mental State Examination: A preliminary study. *Journal of Hong Kong College of Psychiatrists, 4*(Suppl. 2), 25–28.

Chiu, H.F.K, & Zhang, M. (2000). A Chinese view. In J. O'Brien, D. Ames, & A. Burns (Eds.), *Dementia* (2nd ed., pp. 345–352). Oxford, England: Oxford University Press.

Chow, N.W.S. (1987). Western and Chinese ideas of social welfare. *International Social Work, 30*(1), 31–41.

Coen, R., O'Boyle, C., Coakley, D., & Lawlor, B. (1999). Dementia carer education and patient behaviour disturbance. *International Journal of Geriatric Psychiatry, 14,* 302–306.

Cole, R.P., Scott, S., & Skelton-Robinson, M. (2000). The effect of challenging behaviour, and staff support, on the psychological wellbeing of staff working with older adults. *Aging and Mental Health, 4*(4), 359–365.

Diehl, M. (1998). Everyday competence in later life: Current status and future directions. *The Gerontologist, 38*(4), 422–433.

Doody, R.S., Stevens, J.C., Beck, C., Dubinsky, R.M., Kaye, J.A., Gwyther, L., Mohs, R.C., Thal, L.J., Whitehouse, P.J., DeKosky, S.T., & Cummings, J.L. (2001). Practice parameter: Management of dementia (an evidence-based review). *Neurology, 56*(9), 1154–1166.

Elderly Commission. (2001, April 24). *Summary of agenda for the 23rd meeting of the Elderly Commission.* Retrieved from http://www.info.gov.hk/hwb/text/english/advise/summ23.htm

Finkel, S.I., Costa de Silva, J., Cohen, G., Miller, S., & Sartorius, N. (1996). Behavioural and psychological signs and symptoms of dementia: a consensus statement on current knowledge and implications for research and treatment. *International Journal of Psychogeriatrics, 8,* 497–500.

Herrmann, N., & Black, S.E. (2000). Behavioral disturbance in dementia: Will the real treatment please stand up? *Neurology, 55*(9), 1247–1248.

Hong Kong Council of Social Service. (1997). *The study of the needs of elderly people in Hong Kong for residential care and community support services.* Hong Kong, China: Deloitte and Touche Consulting Group.

Hong Kong Hospital Authority. (2000). *Annual Report 1999–2000.* Hong Kong, China: Hong Kong Hospital Authority.

International Psychogeriatric Association. (1998). *Behavioral psychological symptoms of dementia (BPSD) educational pack.* Macclesfield, England: Gardiner-Caldwell Communications.

Kwok, C. (2000). Using Dementia Care Mapping to promote the quality of dementia care. In *Abstract Proceedings of the Hospital Authority Convention* (p. 67). Hong Kong, China: Hong Kong Hospital Authority.

Kwok, C. (2001a). Advancement of dementia care practice by using Dementia Care Mapping. In *Abstract Proceedings of the Nursing Conference, Hospital Authority, Hong Kong* (p. 34). Hong Kong, China: Hong Kong Hospital Authority.

Kwok, C. (2001b). Promotion of activities-focused care for persons with dementia. In *Abstract Proceedings of the Joint Meeting of the International Psychogeriatric Association and the Faculty of Psychiatry of Old Age Royal Australian and New Zealand College of Psychiatrists* (p. 69). Lorne, Australia: C/-ICMS Pty Ltd.

Kwok, C. (2002, April). *Mapping the behaviour: How does it help the nonpharmacological intervention of behaviour and psychological symptoms of dementia?* Presentation at the Hong Kong Alzheimer's Disease Conference 2002, Hong Kong, China.

Lam, L., Tang, W.K., Leung, V., & Chiu, H. (2001). Behavioral profile of Alzheimer's disease in Chinese elderly: A validation study of the Chinese version of the Alzheimer's Disease Behavioral Pathology Rating Scale. *International Journal of Geriatric Psychiatry, 16,* 368–373.

Larson, E.B. (1997). Minimizing excess disability: A common strategy for chronic disease management. *Journal of Geriatric Psychiatry and Neurology, 10,* 49–50.

Lawton, M.P. (1983). Environmental process and other determinants of well-being in older people. *The Gerontologist, 23,* 349–357.

Lee, E.S.H. (2001, November). *Enhancing quality of dementia care: Using Dementia Care Mapping (DCM) as a tool for service audit.* Presentation at the Ninth Annual Congress of Gerontology, Hong Kong Association of Gerontology, Hong Kong, China.

Lin, T.Y., Tseng, W.S., & Yen, E.K. (1995). *Chinese societies and mental health.* New York: Oxford University Press.

Perrin, T. (1998). Single-system methodology: A way forward in dementia care? *British Journal of Occupational Therapy, 61*(10), 448–452.

Rabins, P.V., Lyketsos, C.G., & Steele, C. (1999). *Practical dementia care.* New York: Oxford University Press.

Rogers, J.C., Holm, M.B., Burgio, L.D., Hsu, C., Hardin, M., & McDowell, J. (2000). Excess disability during morning care in nursing home residents with dementia. *International Psychogeriatrics, 12*(2), 267–282.

Sifton, C. (2000). Maximizing the functional abilities of persons with Alzheimer's Disease and Related Dementias. In M.P. Lawton & R.L. Rubinstein (Eds.), *Interventions in dementia Care. Toward improving quality of life* (pp. 11–37). New York: Springer Publishing Co.

Steele, C., Rouner, B., Chase, G.A., & Folstein, M. (1990). Psychiatric symptoms and nursing home placement of patients with Alzheimer's disease. *American Journal of Psychiatry, 147,* 1049–1051.

Tseng, W.S., & Wu, D. (1985). *Chinese culture and mental health.* San Diego: Academic Press.

Working Group on Dementia. (1999). *Report of the Working Group on Dementia.* Retrieved April 3, 2002, from http://www.info.gov.hk/hwb/text/english/legco/w_14_2/demrpt.htm

9

SOCIAL, POLITICAL, AND ECONOMIC CONSIDERATIONS OF DEMENTIA CARE MAPPING

CAROLYN LECHNER

An international phenomenon is occurring as the person-centered approach and Dementia Care Mapping (DCM) are being introduced to those who provide dementia care. Training participants have noted how the classes offer eloquent words and innovative ways of thinking about familiar theories and concepts, which could further help to inform good practice. Kitwood explained that person-centered care is "a fabric woven from two components: ethics and social psychology" (personal communication, March 1998). These theoretical elements shape the course of dementia care on a daily, direct level.

When one crosses over the line from theory into practice, specifically in the practice of DCM, one may also wish to examine from social, economic, and political perspectives the method's applications for dementia care. Certainly, DCM did not evolve as an agent to directly address these issues. On the contrary, it was meant to offer a mode for better examining direct relationships of care and for recognizing and respecting people with dementia as conscious beings.

Nonetheless, it also may be worth observing the impact of these more global disciplines on the method as it continues to develop. Doing so takes the examination of DCM and person-centered care from the microlevel to the macrolevel of observation. It may be worth determining whether an ongoing exploration of DCM from macrolevel areas is a worthwhile endeavor so that understanding of them enhances and does not impede willingness to confront care issues on the microlevel.

By acknowledging the relationship (if any) among the social, political, and economic contexts of care, certain implications for the future can be examined. These areas of concern are on care workers' minds at the beginning of the 21st century, as both the demographics and the needs of elderly individuals make a radical shift. This chapter discusses social, political, and economic aspects of care (as they apply to developed societies) within the context of their relationship to and bearing on the person-centered approach to dementia care and to DCM.

BLAMING THE VICTIM

In *Blaming the Victim,* Ryan (1971) urged the reader to rethink certain commonly held beliefs about U.S. society. He explained how, in an effort to understand why elements of racism and social inequality still percolated under the surface in 1971, he stumbled upon a "mythology" of sorts. In this tradition, the people who most want to improve society may be ultimately responsible for its stasis. Ryan noted, "Good intentions and vigorous actions to improve social conditions are constantly being crippled, sabotaged, and deflected by insidious forces that have already pre-shaped the channels of thought" (p. xiv).

Poverty and racial prejudice are the most prominent themes in Ryan's book, but he briefly recognized public health as a site in which this dynamic can also thrive. Some factions of society choose to put the burden of disease back on diagnosed individuals. In this framework, people diagnosed with dementia would be held responsible for the condition and the burden that they place on their loved ones and their communities.

It is not surprising that in the years since Ryan's treatise was published, educators and experts in the field have echoed Ryan's thinking—but with a dementia-specific twist. Binstock and Murray asked the following:

> Is there a morally relevant difference between one group—be it the aged, the demented, the poor—and any other which justifies unequal treatment in the provision of acute or long-term care? Should different standards of equity be applied to the health care arena than those applied to other spheres of activity in our society? (1991, p. 154)

DCM can play a part in ending this particular blame-the-victim cycle as it relates to the long-term care system and to individuals with dementia. If unfavorable or harmful behavior is recorded during a DCM session and it can be presented insightfully to staff, then each care worker may be able to face personal judgments and prejudices that have no place in the care setting. Again, however, it is the people who want to spearhead improvements the most who are most inclined to blame the victim—they are looking for answers and may not know how to get their arms around the problem.

DCM is presented as a developmental evaluation model, in which those seeking help are asked to confront and consider their own concerns in a new and different way. A skilled mapper helps care workers to find the answers that they are seeking in themselves instead of in the people for whom they care. The answers come from within rather than from an outside victim on whom to lay the burden of the problem.

GLOBAL GRAYING PHENOMENON

One issue that touches older adults on many levels is the demographic shift that has drastic implications for the world in the 21st century. Many pundits and analysts have come to refer to this trend as the "graying" of the world's population. At a rapidly advancing rate, trends show a marked increase in the number of elderly individuals worldwide and a similar decrease in the number of youth.

Experts attribute this trend to three things: 1) medical advances allow more people to live longer, 2) the population born in post–World War II Western societies is moving through middle age, and 3) fertility rates have dropped to the point that meeting the replacement rate is in question (Peterson, 1999). A direct correlation between this graying phenomenon and the composition of DCM, as well as its impact on modes of care improvement and service delivery, may be hard to come by initially. Yet, it definitely indicates that the introduction of the method could not have come at a better time.

As the world attempts to deal with the outcomes of these figures, a backlash against older individuals may need consideration. Some hypothetical questions may emerge as a result of these developments: Is it possible that resentment toward older people and their needs will grow? Will elderly individuals who receive long-term care be exposed to tensions and hostility by their care workers as a result of external and personal circumstances?

Posner wrote, "We do not appear to be genetically programmed to feel as protective toward old people in general; while most people love their parents even when their parents are old, they do so generally with diminished intensity" (1995, p. 203). He suggested that the social value of the older person decreases as he or she continues to age. This leads to a bitter paradox: Technology may increase the life expectancy of each person, but the "reward" that each reaps (in terms of a comforting place in society) may not be worth the effort.

A fundamental negativity toward elderly individuals as a whole may exist, and this may be manifested in the relationship of direct care. In a person-centered approach, one is urged to view and treat the individual with dementia as holistically as possible. Yet, Posner (1995) suggested that even one's own family works against this type of belief system. The result is a sort of stigmatization. The practical applications of DCM in light of these larger societal concepts, therefore, become more visible.

POLITICAL ECONOMY OF AGING

Examining the person-centered approach and DCM from a macro standpoint may appear to be the antithesis of why the methods were designed. It is by exploring systems such as these that one learns how certain structural configurations promote societal responses. For example, from this standpoint, it would be possible to trace the origins and evolution of today's model of dementia care, as well as the stigma and prejudices that too often accompany it.

One theoretical framework that is based on a macrolevel understanding of societal trends is the political economy of aging. In *Critical Perspectives on Aging: The Political and Moral Economy of Growing Old,* Minkler and Cole offered a defining comment: "Political economy provides a valuable framework for understanding how polity, economy, and society shape the conditions, experiences, treatment, and health of older people" (1991, p. 37). In another chapter from the same collection, Estes acknowledged that for many in gerontological fields, the political economy model may not be relevant to those seeking practical applications and improvements:

> The central challenge of the political economy of aging is to understand the character and significance of variations in the treatment of the aged and to relate them to broader societal trends. A major task is to understand how the aging process itself is influenced by the treatment . . . of elders in society. (1991, p. 19)

ECONOMICS OF DEMENTIA

In some ways, using an economic perspective to analyze individuals with dementia places the observer furthest from the principles of person-centered care. Those receiving care produce certain costs, so much analysis is based on exploring how to reduce cost. Can quality of life and quality of care be preserved in such a setting?

Economics seem to play a role in the evolution of DCM as well. Over time, interest in the method has emerged from those who wish to test its efficacy to ensure quality care provision. In addition to changing care practice, many have found that DCM also is an effective means of measuring outcomes. Such innovative uses of DCM may govern the direction of future research regarding the method.

Some experts have noted that people with dementia are disenfranchised; they urge decision makers to include these individuals in future economic forecasting for the older adults. In *Dementia and Aging: Ethics, Values and Policy Choices,* Callahan remarked,

> The peculiar allocation problem we face with the dementias is that the features they display tend to bring out the worst in the . . . system, and the demands they place on the system—especially for personal care and social services—are just those we have most commonly resisted. (1991, p. 142)

In another chapter of the same collection, Binstock and Murray (1991) recalled Callahan's earlier thoughts about a somewhat controversial concept that had once received a lot of attention: rationing acute care services to more adequately meet the population's need for long-term care. At one time, Callahan proposed that if decision makers continued in their then-current direction, age and cognitive impairment might become criteria for the provision or refusal of long-term care. Binstock and Murray (and, later, Callahan himself) ultimately believed that such a plan is "poorly developed" and could not succeed.

Callahan, Binstock and Murray, and many others questioned yet another paradigm that applies to the economic delivery of services to people with dementia. In this model, the traditional top-down approach, policymakers are the elite few who make decisions for the many. The model is challenged by the bottom-up approach, which involves decision making at the grass roots level and by the people receiving care. The parallels between this model and Kitwood's (1997) "old culture/new culture" paradigm are easily visible.

Callahan stated that for those with dementia to be recognized, "It will require a revolution in our thinking and our practices" (1991, p. 142). Callahan further recommended that policy makers change priorities and look for a new philosophy of care. This recommendation suggests that DCM would be a welcome presence in a new culture of health care. As of 2002, economic support for people with dementia appears to be governed by a concept that is discussed in the next section, biomedicalization.

BIOMEDICALIZATION OF AGING

The concept *biomedicalization of aging* has become an area of concern for those with dementia. By consigning elderly individuals to a management system under the auspices of a rigidly medical model, an entire group within society can be efficiently handled, leaving leaders more time to focus on other issues. Estes and Binney (1991) described how biomedicalization of aging takes place on a thinking level and on a practice/care level. Biomedicalization has already had a profound, worldwide impact on service delivery to older adults as well as to people with cognitive impairments.

Kitwood also explored the implications of biomedicalization and subsequently utilized the term often in his own writing. He classified the medical model of care as the standard paradigm, which governs and informs the standard of dementia care throughout the world. Kitwood created a table (1997, p. 136) that contrasted the medical and social models so that care workers could see the differences for themselves.

Kitwood (1997) argued that the progressive cognitive impairment of dementia should not be ignored or denied. Rather, he believed that it is one of many factors that contributes to the overall experience of dementia. Kuhn, Ortigara, and Kasayka wrote,

> Kitwood's theory about dementia . . . [is about] more than a neurologic phenomenon resulting in cognitive impairments that can also lead to social and psychologic disintegration. He argued that disintegration occurs mainly as a result of the destructive social environment [in which people with dementia] find themselves. (2000, p. 8)

Kitwood (1997) suggested that an exclusively medical model does not make sense. It results in families and care workers waiting anxiously for a dementia cure and continuing to suffer in their current day-to-day experiences. Via DCM, people are realizing that in the meantime, they can change the way that they perceive and care for people with dementia.

Like Kitwood, Robertson suggested that an alternative construction of Alzheimer's disease exists: "Disease is a social construct, that is, a way of looking at human experience, a way of organizing 'reality'" (1991, p. 137). By compartmentalizing dementia into a tidy medical package, a certain degree of responsibility is avoided. Kitwood refused to bow to the medical construct of dementia. He wrote that "one of the most encouraging signs in recent years is that at last people with dementia are being recognized as having true subjectivity" (1997, p. 70). Kitwood explained how he learned what people with dementia need: He took the focus of inquiry from the macrolevel back to the microlevel.

OLD CULTURE VERSUS NEW CULTURE

Kitwood (1997) shared the idea that dementia care is in the process of a massive paradigm shift: Courageous pioneers are leaving the "old culture" behind in favor of the promise of a "new culture." He delineated the relationship of old versus new and offered his suggestions regarding how each facility can make the shift. According to Kitwood, these changes must take place within each individual care worker, but this is best achieved via organizational change.

Kitwood's model for DCM also places great value on communication within the realm of the change process. Based on a pluralistic approach, in which as many points of view are acknowledged as possible, DCM seeks to engage change on a global organizational level. Kitwood (personal communication, March 1998) noted that contradictions and incompatibilities will emerge as a result of this approach but that even these elements add richness to the ultimate result of the change process.

Thomas (1996) came to a similar crossroads, when he believed that the old culture no longer sufficed for the people for whom he cared. Thomas created the Eden Alternative, a program and philosophy that is meant to transform a nursing facility from an institutional setting to a more nurturing, home-like one. Thomas explained that including gardens, animals, and children conveys a sense of vibrancy and livelihood to residents, who may be confronting questions about their validity and worth.

Some parallels exist between the visions of Kitwood and Thomas. Kitwood used language that incorporated the concepts of old and new cultures; Thomas spoke of revolutions within the care setting. Specifically, Thomas mentioned two revolutions that result from "Edenization." The first is the palpable one: The nursing home setting is physically transformed. In the second one, values, beliefs, and attitudes throughout the spectrum of care are challenged and sometimes revised. Thus, much like Kitwood, Thomas made provisions for the short and the long term.

In addition to DCM and Edenization, other campaigns are moving forward to improve the quality of care and levels of well-being for people with dementia who live in formal settings. For example, the National Citizens'

Coalition for Nursing Home Reform (NCCNHR) was formed in Washington, D.C., in 1975, during a gathering for the National Gray Panthers' Long Term Care Action Project. Over the years, the coalition and its founder Elma Holder have committed themselves to the improvement of care offered in U.S. nursing facilities.

NCCNHR played a major role in the development of the Omnibus Budget Reconciliation Act (OBRA) of 1987 (PL 100-203), known as the Nursing Home Reform Act, and it has subsequently worked toward full implementation of the law. NCCNHR committed itself to providing "information and leadership on federal and state regulatory and legislative policy development and models and strategies to improve care and life for residents of nursing homes and other long term care facilities" (NCCNHR, 2001a). Over time, NCCNHR has taken on the challenge of upholding the laws it helped to create, from monitoring Medicaid entitlements to educating U.S. officials about the direct care level issues, such as the use of physical and chemical restraints.

In 2001, the NCCNHR, along with 30 other organizations, endorsed *The Nurse Staffing Crisis in Nursing Homes: A Consensus Statement of the Campaign for Quality Care.* In an ongoing overlap of the values and goals of DCM, this document outlined the dilemma that long-term care nurses face in terms of quality care provision and residents' well-being. The document also provided potential directions for finding solutions.

Further exploration of these and other issues appears imminent over the next several years. The Pioneer Network is another U.S. organization that has emerged with the intention of improving quality of care and increasing well-being for people with dementia and others who reside in long-term care settings. This organization's primary commitment is reconsidering and reshaping how long-term care is provided.

In 2001, the Pioneer Network held a conference, which DCM representatives attended to determine if and how DCM might play a part in bringing about this paradigm shift. DCM advocates and members of the Pioneer Network clearly share a common language. The Pioneers espouse the concept of "culture change," and its goals and values are consistent with Kitwood's design for a new culture of care (1997, p. 135).

These organizations exist to provide education and resources to those interested in change—specifically, an improvement in the care that is provided in long-term care settings at the beginning of the 21st century. Perhaps because of their specific applicability to the American political and economic systems, these agencies have achieved a visibility and influence that DCM has yet to attain. These organizations have access to and understanding of their role in the policy process.

ROLE OF POLICY

The need for innovative changes in U.S. public policy was a prominent focus of the World Alzheimer's Congress, which took place in Washington, D.C. during the summer of 2000. In conjunction with the World Alzheimer's Congress, the American Alzheimer's Association released an action plan entitled *2000 Federal Legislative Priorities.* In addition to identifying new ways to support family care workers, the document advocates a search for new methods of service delivery "in ways that protect consumers without overmedicalizing care and inflating costs, and to hold providers accountable for quality" (Alzheimer's Association, p. 3).

Some health care leaders want to reexamine the care worker system to strengthen it. As far back as 1989, experts noted the dynamics of the settings into which nursing aides and people with dementia are placed. Tellis-Nayak and Tellis-Nayak described the situation as "two parties, both powerless, little respected, and hardly recognized by society and made to face each other in a difficult setting not of their own making" (1989, p. 312).

Just as DCM urges the care worker to recognize the voice of the resident, it can be used to hear and honor the voice of the professional care worker as well. One newspaper article written during the World Alzheimer's Congress explored the role of the nursing aide in relation to the role of the individual with dementia. One care worker stated that "the process made him feel more integral to his patient's lives, while making him a more sensitive caregiver" (Allen, 2000, p. S1).

Similarly, McConnell and Riggs (1999) of the Alzheimer's Association listed some recommendations in response to a litany of policy challenges that Alzheimer's disease presents. They wrote, "Alzheimer's care providers need special training to understand the disease, to deal with behaviors that may be frustrating, frightening and even dangerous, and to recognize health problems that need prompt attention" (p. 72). DCM offers a viable solution for the care worker who wants to gain a better understanding of Alzheimer's disease and the person diagnosed with it, as well as how to best communicate with that individual.

Van Kleunen and Wilner echoed these sentiments, noting that "the quality of the care received by long-term care consumers is directly related to the quality of the job offered to the paraprofessionals who deliver that care on a day-to-day basis" (2000, p. 116). Furthermore, they proposed that standards for paraprofessionals become more stringent, not only to ensure quality but also to retain and promote those care workers in the workforce. Participants in the basic DCM certification course learn that for the person-centered approach to pervade a facility, it has to be offered by care workers to residents, shared between care workers, and demonstrated by administrators to care workers.

To explore the tool's global potential, representatives from the United Kingdom and the United States presented an evaluation of U.K. and U.S. settings that use DCM. The Innes and Lechner (2000) compared data from care settings in both countries and identified the unique cultural implications that DCM may have across cultures. As interest in DCM expands to additional countries, maintaining cultural sensitivity—in keeping with Kitwood's core beliefs in personhood (1997)—is essential.

Furthermore, as DCM continues to grow in popularity worldwide, it may also have to evolve into a method that can meet the needs of those who receive care outside of formal long-term care settings. DCM's creators and contributors to DCM's success have revisited the practicalities of the method and the person-centered approach that accompanies it. These individuals have renewed their belief that the underlying philosophy of the person-centered approach markedly alters the culture of care, regardless of where it is offered.

CONCLUSION

An exploration of social, economic, and political considerations of DCM can yield further understanding of the method and its effects. In turn, grasping these issues helps policy makers navigate the economic and political terrain of improving long-term care and, specifically, dementia care. Yet, the two elements that Kitwood has cited—ethics and social psychology—are still at the method's core and inform everything else.

As this chapter has noted, the macrolevel model may have an impact on perceptions of dementia around the world, taking the concept of dementia itself to a new level. A macrolevel examination of DCM can explore how the method's presence in the realms of economics and politics affects people with dementia. It seems that a macrolevel exploration of person-centered care entails a paradoxical relationship, however, as the focus of person-centered care is fairly self-explanatory. Therefore, although it is intriguing to consider the relationships between DCM and the social sciences, including economics and politics, it is paramount to remember that, as Kitwood (1997) said, "the person comes first."

REFERENCES

Allen, J.A. (2000, August 5). Alzheimer's care crisis. *The Los Angeles Times,* p. S1.
Alzheimer's Association (2000). *2000 federal legislative priorities.* Retrieved October 2001 from http://www.alz.org/involved/advocacy/fed_longterm.htm#Meeting

Binstock, R.H., & Murray, T.H. (1991). The politics of developing appropriate care for dementia. In R.H. Binstock, S.G. Post, & P.J. Whitehouse (Eds.), *Dementia and aging: Ethics, values, and policy choices* (pp. 153–170). Baltimore: The Johns Hopkins University Press.

Callahan, D. (1991). Dementia and appropriate care: Allocating scarce resources. In R.H. Binstock, S.G. Post, & P.J. Whitehouse (Eds.), *Dementia and aging: Ethics, values, and policy choices* (pp. 141–152). Baltimore: The Johns Hopkins University Press.

Estes, C.L. (1991). The new political economy of aging: Introduction and critique. In M. Minkler & C.L. Estes (Eds.), *Critical perspectives on aging: The political and moral economy of growing old* (pp. 19–36). Amityville, NY: Baywood Publishing Company.

Estes, C.L., & Binney, E.A. (1991). The biomedicalization of aging: Dangers and dilemmas. In M. Minkler & C.L. Estes (Eds.), *Critical perspectives on aging: The political and moral economy of growing old* (pp. 117–134). Amityville, NY: Baywood Publishing Company.

Innes, A., & Lechner, C. (2000). High-quality dementia care across cultures: An international evaluation of settings using the Dementia Care Mapping method. *The World Alzheimer Congress 2000 Proceedings Book, Session F13.* Washington, DC: Alzheimer's Disease and Related Disorders Association.

Kitwood, T. (1997). *Dementia reconsidered: The person comes first.* Buckingham, England: Open University Press.

Kuhn, D., Ortigara, A., & Kasayka, R.E. (2000). Dementia Care Mapping: An innovative tool to measure person-centered care. *Alzheimer's Care Quarterly, 1*(3), 7–15.

McConnell, S., & Riggs, J. (1999, Fall). The policy challenges of Alzheimer's disease. *Generations, 23*(3), 69–74.

Minkler, M., & Cole, T.R. (1991). Political and moral economy. In M. Minkler & C.L. Estes (Eds.), *Critical perspectives on aging: The political and moral economy of growing old* (pp. 37–49). Amityville, NY: Baywood Publishing Company.

Minkler, M., & Estes, C.L. (Eds.). (1991). *Critical perspectives on aging: The political and moral economy of growing old.* Amityville, NY: Baywood Publishing Company.

National Citizens' Coalition for Nursing Home Reform (NCCNHR). (2001a). *About NCCNHR.* Retrieved October 2001 from http://www.nccnhr.org/static_pages/about.cfm

National Citizens' Coalition for Nursing Home Reform (NCCNHR). (2001b, June 26). *The nursing staff crisis in nursing homes: A consensus statement of the Campaign for Quality Care (March 14, 2000).* Retrieved April 2002 from http://www.nccnhr.org/govpolicy/51_162_701.cfm

Omnibus Budget Reconciliation Act (OBRA) of 1987 (PL 100-203).

Peterson, P.G. (1999). *Gray dawn: How the coming age wave will transform America—and the world.* New York: Random House.

Posner, R.A. (1995). *Aging and old age.* Chicago: University of Chicago Press.

Robertson, A. (1991). The politics of Alzheimer's disease: A case study in apocalyptic demography. In M. Minkler & C.L. Estes (Eds.), *Critical perspectives on aging: The political and moral economy of growing old* (pp. 135–149). Amityville, NY: Baywood Publishing Company.

Ryan, W. (1971). *Blaming the victim.* New York: Vintage & Anchor Books.

Tellis-Nayak, V., & Tellis-Nayak, M. (1989). Quality of care and the burden of two cultures: When the world of the nurse's aide enters the world of the nursing home. *The Gerontologist, 29*(3), 307–313.

Thomas, W.H. (1996). *Life worth living: How someone you love can still enjoy life in a nursing home.* Acton, MA: VanderWyk & Burnham.

Van Kleunen, A., & Wilner, M.A. (2000). Who will care for mother tomorrow? *Journal of Aging and Social Policy, 11*(2/3), 115–126.

IV

FUTURE USES OF
DEMENTIA CARE
MAPPING

10

LESSONS FOR COGNITIVE
DISABILITY SERVICES

MICHELLE PERSAUD

Care services often struggle to assess quality of care. The problems faced in dementia and cognitive disability care services mirror each other, as the people receiving care are often unable to articulate opinions. The work of Kitwood and Bredin was an innovation, with its attempt to address the difficulties faced by evaluators of services (see Bradford Dementia Group, 1997).

The very nature of person-centered care has been at the forefront of disability care services since the work of Nirje, Bank-Mikkleson, and Wolfensberger in the 1960s and 1970s (Flynn & Nitsch, 1980). Kitwood's concept of *malignant social psychology* bears many similarities to Wolfensberger's theory of normalization. When discussing the person-centered approach to care with a colleague who has a dementia care background, it became apparent that this approach was similar to that used in services for people with cognitive disabilities. Therefore, it seemed appropriate to investigate whether disability professionals could benefit from using the work of their dementia care colleagues. Although Dementia Care Mapping (DCM) was designed for use with people with dementia, it is worthy of investigation for other client groups. This chapter discusses the first research of its kind on using DCM in the disabilities field.

Many people with cognitive disabilities in the United Kingdom live in residential care settings provided by government authorities, nonprofit organizations, and private groups. Testing care quality is fraught with difficulties, as third-party opinion often becomes the focus of any evaluation (Hoyes, 1990; Stanley & Roy, 1988; Thomas, Felce, de Kock, Saxby, & Repp, 1986). In the 20th century, there was a heavy reliance on evaluation methods that concentrated on quantifiable and tangible aspects of care (e.g., environmental aspects of facilities). Wolfensberger and Glenn argued that, traditionally, services were not fully evaluated because managers believed that it was inappropriate to put "price tags" on services that directly benefit human beings (1975, p. 4). They also argued that the lack of appropriate measurement scales, devices, or systems exacerbated the status quo situation of nonevaluation. They asserted, "Too often we have made the quantifiable important instead of the important quantifiable" (p. 4).

A research project was developed to test the question, "How useful is DCM for assessing quality of care in the environment of a hospital that serves people with cognitive disabilities?" This project developed from an awareness of the already robust research agenda within the dementia field (e.g., Innes & Surr, 2001) and a recognition of the similar issues facing service providers in the disabilities and dementia care fields. The project also completed the requirements prescribed by Bradford University to ensure appropriate application and use of DCM (Innes, Capstick, & Surr, 2000).

The work's success depended on the methods used, and it became apparent that an established, respected form of research in nursing—ethnonursing—lent itself to the task. One of the greatest benefits from using this type of research is that it provides, in Leininger's words "detailed accounts of events, situations and circumstances that are usually difficult to discover by other research methods" (1985, p. 40). The intention for the process was to use an empirical, experimental, "have a go at it" approach. This way, the method could be used, results could be gathered, and experiences could be reflected on regarding how the project felt and worked in practice. In one sense, this application of DCM could be described as a clinical trial—that is, testing something in a clinical setting. In the context of this work, *experimental* means trying something as opposed to testing cause and effect (Polit & Hungler, 1999).

For the purposes of the study, a convenience design was chosen (Polit & Hungler, 1999). To reflect the variety of disabilities represented in a local hospital, three residential care areas were chosen in which to conduct observations. In total, 22 people were observed, representing 96% of the population living in the target areas. The age range was 20–63 years, and all participants had severe cognitive impairments, as defined by England's 1983 Mental Health Act (Gostin, 1983). None of the participants had a diagnosis of dementia; however, many had communication difficulties. This factor allowed testing of the assertion that DCM could evaluate the care they received— something that they could not describe for themselves.

Criteria for success needed to be selected. It was determined that the project's success would be demonstrated by observing DCM's workability in a cognitive disability care setting. In other words, the project would address the questions "How applicable is the method?" "What are the strengths of using it out of context?" and "What are the limitations?" The next three sections address these questions in detail.

APPLICABILITY TO COGNITIVE DISABILITY SERVICES

DCM was designed solely for use in dementia care settings, and its evaluation codes have been refined after thousands of observation hours. Twenty-three codes, plus one for indistinguishable behaviors, are available to the observer. These compose what DCM calls Behaviour Category Codes (BCC; see Table 1 in the Introduction for a complete list of codes). When DCM is applied in a dementia care setting, observed behaviors are distinctive of dementia and stable. Kitwood (1997) asserted that the emerging and testable social psychology of dementia is closely linked to DCM. This psychology would allow a clear account of the experience of dementia. All of DCM's key constructs arise from this psychology, and he purports DCM to be a construct-type method (i.e., a method that identifies the nature, essence, and underlying attributes of the phenomenon under study).

Again, Kitwood (1997) stated that dementia has a testable social psychology, which is supported by how easily behaviors can be interpreted in a dementia setting. The testable nature of dementia makes it easy to observe and interpret the behaviors of those who have it (Robinson & Reed, 1998). The experience proved that although there is a wealth of knowledge about the nature, essence, and underlying attributes of cognitive disabilities, there is also a tremendous variety of behaviors for which the DCM coding was not sufficient or appropriate.

The DCM code *I* (Intellectual—reading, doing another intellectual activity) can mean reading books or magazines. During the observations, it was observed that a few of the participants enjoyed "reading" catalogs. This situation illustrated a difficulty with interpretation. If a staff member was actually sitting with the participant, reading to him or her and carrying out an intellectual-type activity (e.g., a question-and-answer session), then it would be appropriate to code this behavior as I. If the participant was just enjoying the pictures, however, then coding the event is problematic.

Difficulty with interpretation also occurred when behaviors exhibited in a dementia setting took on a different connotation in the cognitive disability care setting. For example, DCM describes a person's walking within his or her care area as a Type 2 behavior (behavior that does not involve anyone other than the individual). With its potential to be solitary in nature and lacking in purpose, such behavior is not usually considered positive.

Within the cognitive disability care environment, this behavior took on two completely different aspects. On the one hand, most of the participants tended to walk in the same areas or on the same spot repeatedly. In this sense, the behavior was repetitive and self-stimulatory and, as such, could have been coded as a W (Withstanding—self-stimulatory behavior). On the other hand, the behavior was viewed positively for people who also had physical disabilities and mobility problems. For them, walking—even without a purpose—facilitated independence. Therefore, this behavior could be coded within the J (Joints—participating in exercise) category if the nature of the activity indicated exercise of some type.

The positive nature of a behavior can also be reflected in Well- or Ill-Being (WIB) scores. One problem for observers, however, was when much time was spent in the activity. For Type 2 solitary behavior, some of the behavior codes have a degeneration rule attached, which is reflected in the WIB score as "noninteraction." Say that a person is sitting down, staring at the floor; this would be considered a C (Cool—socially uninvolved) behavior. If the person remains in this state for 30 continuous minutes, then his or her WIB score drops (e.g., from $+1$ to -1). After another 30 minutes, it degenerates again from -1 to -3; then, 30 minutes later, it drops to a -5 score.

K (Kum and go—walking or standing independently) does not carry the degeneration rule. Therefore, the observers believed that the solitary nature of the pacing was not adequately reflected in a person's WIB score. In one instance, it was noted that a participant paced the same corridor for almost 6 hours, but the WIB score remained within a positive domain. The coding fails in this area. This degeneration rule problem is also true of codes Y (Yourself—talking to oneself or an imagined friend) and W (Withstanding—self-stimulatory behavior). Both behaviors are frequent in people with cognitive disabilities and, thus, are scored consistently in the observations.

This study also yielded a surprising finding: recognition of mappers' need for support. Carrying out long, intensive periods of observation, particularly watching care delivery, can have a profound effect on an individual. The whole process calls into question one's own practice as a care worker. Intense, mixed emotions can be experienced, especially when one is observing an area that demonstrates questionable or deficient care delivery. All of the mappers involved in the project recognized this factor and expressed a need for support following a period of mapping. This is true of both cognitive disability and dementia care settings.

STRENGTHS OF USING DEMENTIA CARE MAPPING FOR PEOPLE WITH COGNITIVE DISABILITIES

The efficacy of DCM in cognitive disability care settings is debatable. Compared with dementia care settings, effectiveness is limited. Yet, if the intent of using DCM is to highlight areas of deficiency or good practice in care delivery, then it has been very effective in cognitive disability care settings—regardless of coding problems.

DCM facilitated the collection of rich, detailed data. All relevant scores and indices could be computed. Both individual and group care summaries were completed, along with a final report that had recommendations for each area of the care setting. In this sense, the method was just as efficient used out of the dementia care context.

In addition, applying DCM to care facilities for people with cognitive disabilities efficiently supplied staff with hard data on the types and frequency of behaviors in which participants were engaged. Particularly relevant was that in all three observation areas, A (Articulation—interacting verbally) behaviors were virtually nonexistent. Care workers should strive to increase A behaviors to enhance individuals' emotional well-being. Given that cognitive disability care environments usually have philosophies that embrace emotional support and well-being, this aspect completely surprised many staff who would not have believed that the interaction levels were so low unless presented with hard evidence. In the three areas mapped, the percentage of time that care workers spent interacting with participants was 38% for Area 1, 12% for Area 2, and 2% for Area 3. These results indicate the need to address the cultural values of care within the environments. Questions about philosophies and attitudes clearly must be asked, as the results demonstrate a "warehousing" and task orientation to care delivery.

The data highlighted one particular phenomenon. In all of the areas chosen within the sample, student nurses were on duty. The data showed that in all instances, the care workers tended to busy themselves with physical care or similar tasks (e.g., making beds). It was apparent that none of them actually sat down and talked with participants. Discussion with the other observers revealed two possible reasons for this finding:

1. The students in a clinical placement have to fulfill certain objectives and, therefore, keep busy in an attempt to obtain a good postplacement appraisal. This may be a rather cynical viewpoint, but it is worthy of consideration.

2. The students have not been taught how to work with people who require long-term care and may not be able to give substantial verbal feedback. Caregiving in these situations has particular stresses and strains, and the skills for sustaining interaction in these circumstances are not necessarily learned quickly or in a classroom. Roberts and Obholzer asserted that "obsessional routines of care can serve to protect patients from carers [care workers]," who are weighed down by the responsibility of caring for people with permanent conditions (1994, p. 83).

It is clear from the data that care workers avoided engagement with the participants. Even from this small sample, it is evident that the education, training, and support of students in placement situations must be considered. If these issues are not addressed early in professional instruction, avoidance and the subsequent task-oriented culture may continue.

The debate about DCM's efficacy for people with cognitive disabilities will undoubtedly continue, but the most significant finding of this research is that a huge gap still exists between care philosophies and care practices. Cultural change in relation to care delivery appears necessary. To endorse this statement, the results in all observed areas overwhelmingly demonstrated the task-oriented nature of care delivery. Although staff may report that their care focuses on residents' emotional needs and well-being, the data produced do not substantiate this claim. DCM has provided the vehicle for driving change and, as such, is highly effective in the cognitive disability care field. This statement is supported by the words of Leininger, founder and leader of the transcultural nursing field: "[The] unique characteristic of nursing is care, and to discover what best defines care requires an array of qualitative methods to tease out and grasp its hidden and culturally based values" (1985, p. 22).

Time to simply sit and observe for 8 hours is not usually afforded in health care settings. Consequently, DCM gave detailed, rich data, from which staff could benefit by learning how to improve care delivery. For example, a staff nurse was completely shocked to learn from the data that a man in her care had not been talked to for 8 hours! Usually, people are so busy getting on with everything that details slip away and are missed. Effectiveness, then, is a matter of debate that depends on one's point of view and the findings available at this early stage of research.

LIMITATIONS OF USING DEMENTIA CARE MAPPING FOR PEOPLE WITH COGNITIVE DISABILITIES

Efficiency considerations must address resource issues. A significant investment must be maintained if DCM is to be carried out appropriately in both dementia and cognitive disability care settings. Individual service groups decide whether the potential for improvements in care delivery outweighs the cost of training and releasing staff.

The Hawthorne effect (positive change in people who know that they are being observed) is an area of concern regarding the efficiency of DCM data collection for people with cognitive disabilities. Polit and Hungler asserted that a "double Hawthorne effect" may be present in the nursing field, as staff *and* patients alter their behavior because of the observer's presence (1999, p. 185). Kitwood defended this assertion by arguing that care workers are usually far too busy to do anything out of the ordinary. This position does not need to be defended regarding participants with dementia, as the nature of dementia often blocks any impact of the observer's presence.

Within cognitive disability care facilities, however, a stranger can have a profound impact on residents. This project's mapping team found this assertion to be true. Many participants in one of the groups had displayed autistic behavior. While observing in an area, it became apparent that one participant was deliberately waiting to see whether an observer was watching him. This developed into a situation in which the participant began to actively seek the mapper. It was clear that her presence had an effect on his behavior and, therefore, the map scores. Data reliability in this instance is questionable. People with autism or autistic tendencies fear and dislike change. Howlin stated,

> Although, as they grow older, many people with autism come to accept and even enjoy greater variation in their lives, they may continue to resist changes in particular settings, or in certain aspects of their environment; unpredictable changes, too, frequently provoke considerable distress. (1997, p. 101)

On reflection, a judgment error was made in the sample choice. It undoubtedly affected the data for that particular participant, whose behavior differed as a result of observer presence.

One possible solution is to have the observers spend time in the care areas prior to mapping so that residents become familiar with them. The drawback of this approach is the issue of resources. Mapping entails a high fiscal cost without devoting extra time to familiarization within environments. Given the recruitment and retention problems that caregiving services face at the beginning of the 21st century, it is highly unlikely that this solution would be viable or acceptable.

As noted previously, DCM's efficiency in collecting the data for cognitive disabilities care settings has been partially proven. BCC has proven to be the most efficient, especially in demonstrating the types of behaviors in which people are engaged. It is recognized, however, that modifications are necessary to completely tailor the codes to this environment.

DCM proves to be significantly less efficient in the WIB scoring for people with cognitive disabilities. Major adjustments are required not only in the scoring system (i.e., in the degeneration rules), but also in aligning the scores to be more appropriate for this setting. To clarify this point, the overall scores in all three areas made it apparent that positive group WIB scores did not always reflect what was actually observed. Again, consider the example of the participant who paced a corridor for 6 hours without interaction. Overall, however, the DCM method has shown itself to be useable in cognitive disability care settings.

CONCLUSION

Using DCM in cognitive disability care settings has great potential, as demonstrated by the rich, detailed data it yielded in the study described in this chapter. Because of the first experiences of doing the work and the free access to previously "out of bounds" areas, people are more comfortable with mappers' presence.

DCM has great potential for these settings if the method's BCC and WIB scores are redefined. Making BCC more appropriate for people with cognitive disabilities and realigning WIB scoring to accurately reflect observers' experiences are certainly viable propositions. Achieving these goals would also give DCM enormous potential for use in services for people who have cognitive disabilities *and* dementia. Demographic trends indicate that like the rest of the population, people with cognitive disabilities are living longer and, therefore, have an increased risk of developing dementia (Moss, Lambe, & Hogg, 1998).

The greatest potential for applying DCM to other settings lies in the fact that it has proven to be useable outside of the domain for which it was designed. An important aspect of this study was the experience of being a participant observer. Having the time to observe and score within a structured framework focuses the researcher's mind and frees him or her from all other responsibilities except observation. This facility enables the emergence of a rich and detailed picture, which is ordinarily missed in the daily business of caregiving. The impact of "just" watching care delivery is enormous; at times, it leads the observer to question why certain obvious things have not been highlighted before. It stimulates questions about change and culture as well as about how improvements can be made and—more important—sustained. Support and supervision issues are raised, too.

It is hoped that the future potential for this work can be developed. The purpose of caregiving services is to improve care for clients. To do this successfully, staff also have to be cared for and supported. As Kitwood asserted,

> The way in which an organisation treats its staff will be reflected in the DCM data. Staff who are undervalued, or disempowered, or who are working near to the threshold of burnout, will tend to disengage as soon as essential tasks have been carried out, and malignant social psychology is likely to be common. When staff are properly supported, and enabled to flourish in the workplace, the general social psychology of the care environment will be of a much higher quality. (1997, p. 8)

Time, commitment, and resources are required to bring about change. Yet, with motivation and a willingness to learn from colleagues in other care fields, anything is achievable.

The experience of completing this study was illuminating. The benefits have already been demonstrated through improvements to care delivery within the areas that were mapped. When embarking on the work, it was hoped that the method would prove successful. Guarded optimism was tempered with the reality that DCM might not be viable in a cognitive disability care setting. Surprisingly, DCM yielded detailed and rich observations, and the method transferred to an alternative care setting. Work must continue to develop this unique tool into something that the cognitive disability services field can utilize and learn from in the future.

REFERENCES

Bradford Dementia Group. (1997). *Evaluating dementia care: The DCM method* (7th ed.). Bradford, England: University of Bradford.

Flynn, R.J., & Nitsch, K.E. (Eds.). (1980). *Normalization, social integration, and community services.* Baltimore: University Park Press.

Gostin, L. (1983). *A practical guide to mental health law. The Mental Health Act 1983 and related legislation.* London: MIND.

Howlin, P. (1997). *Autism: Preparing for adulthood.* London: Routledge.

Hoyes, L. (1990). *Promoting an ordinary life: A checklist for assessing residential care for people with learning difficulties.* Bristol, England: University of Bristol, School for Advanced Urban Studies.

Innes, A., Capstick, A., & Surr, C. (2000). Mapping out the framework. *Journal of Dementia Care, 8*(2), 20–21.

Innes, A., & Surr, C. (2001). Measuring the well-being of people with dementia living in formal care settings: The use of Dementia Care Mapping. *Aging & Mental Health, 5*(3), 258–268.

Kitwood, T. (1997). *Dementia reconsidered: The person comes first.* Buckingham, England: Open University Press.

Leininger, M. (Ed.). (1985). *Qualitative research methods in nursing.* Philadelphia: W.B. Saunders Company.

Moss, S., Lambe, L., & Hogg, J. (1998). *Ageing matters: Pathways for older people with a learning disability.* Wolverhampton, England: British Institute of Learning Disabilities.

Polit, D., & Hungler, B. (1999). *Nursing research: Principles and methods* (6th ed.). Philadelphia: Lippincott Williams & Wilkins.

Roberts, Z., & Obholzer, A. (Eds.). (1994). *The unconscious at work: Individual and organisational stress in the human services.* London: Routledge.

Robinson, D., & Reed, V. (Eds.). (1998). *The A to Z of social research jargon.* Aldershot, England: Ashgate Publishing.

Stanley, B., & Roy, A. (1988). Evaluating the quality of life of people with mental handicaps: A social validation study. *Mental Handicap Research, 1*(2), 197–210.

Thomas, M., Felce, D., de Kock, U., Saxby, H., & Repp, A. (1986). The activity of staff and profoundly mentally handicapped adults in residential settings of different sizes. *British Journal of Mental Subnormality, 32,* 82–92.

Wolfensberger, W., & Glenn, L. (1975). *Program Analysis of Service Systems (PASS): A method for the quantitative evaluation of human services* (3rd ed.). Toronto: National Institute on Mental Retardation.

11

FUTURE CHALLENGES
FOR DEMENTIA
CARE MAPPING

DAWN BROOKER

The following vision of the future is colored by my experience of Dementia Care Mapping (DCM) developments as of 2002 and by my knowledge of key players and forces within the field of dementia care. I am indebted to those in the DCM community who share their ideas freely, and much of this chapter's material is expounded in the transcripts of the DCM Think Tank (Brooker & Rogers, 2001). My vision for the future within this chapter is limited to the next 3–5 years. Beyond that, much of today's concepts about high-quality dementia care will probably seem crass and outdated.

As a trainee clinical psychologist, I observed a planning meeting for a new learning disabilities community unit following the closure of a large institution. As part of its design, the chair of the planning team advocated building a bomb into the foundation that would destroy the building after 10 years, preventing people with learning disabilities from having to endure what would be, by then, outdated services. These were wise words. Of course, 20 years later, the unit is still standing—but now it is a nursing facility for people with dementia! Maybe evaluation and assessment tools, like buildings, should have a limited shelf life. There may be an essence of DCM that lives on

147

past the next 5–10 years, but the tool itself has to evolve significantly if it is to continue pushing the boundaries of best practice.

MAINTAINING AN ETHICAL FRAMEWORK

Since 2001, I have been the first Strategic Lead for DCM employed specifically by Bradford Dementia Group to focus on the development of DCM. As this book shows, DCM has reached a size and organizational complexity that necessitates such a role. My job of Strategic Lead includes development of the method itself through research and experience, ensuring that DCM training equips people to use the tool reliably and that those who are using the method are adequately supported. Interest in DCM is worldwide and, as a result, my job also includes overseeing the international development and helping the various countries set up DCM training and evaluation in a safe manner.

Safety may seem an odd term to use in respect to DCM. After all, it could be seen as just another evaluation or audit tool that should be freely available for all to use. Since its inception by Kitwood and Bredin, DCM has always been rooted in an ethical framework of person-centered care that promotes the well-being of people with dementia, their families, and their care workers. The complex structures set up around the learning and application of the method are in place to ensure that DCM is used within this ethical framework (Innes, Capstick, & Surr, 2000). At its heart, DCM is a powerful tool that investigates the interpersonal relationships of those with dementia and those who care for them. This is a delicate area of human endeavor. Clumsy feedback or misinterpretations of observations can create emotional distress for staff and, in turn, lead to increased ill-being for care recipients.

DCM is a complex method that requires skill and care in its teaching, its implementation within organizations, and its use in research if all involved are to be treated in a person-centered way and the ethical framework is to be maintained. These structures will likely remain in place, but they will evolve as the use of DCM becomes even more widespread. As of 2002, the international DCM community is centered at the Bradford Dementia Group, where Kitwood developed it and, arguably, where the greatest amount of expertise in using DCM lies. As worldwide experience and expertise is gained, the challenge will be in building structures that can ensure that DCM continues to be used within an ethical framework. The flip side to this challenge is ensuring that DCM is available, in as timely a manner as possible, to all who wish to use it. The structures put in place to protect the vulnerable should not be so bureaucratic that they prohibit the tool's use and development.

FIT FOR PURPOSE

As of 2002, DCM is used for many purposes in different service contexts. The challenge is to ensure that the method is fit for the purpose for which it is being used and, possibly, to adapt the method to ensure its fitness for these different purposes. The most common use of DCM is to improve the standards of person-centered care by a repeated cycle of developmental evaluations (Brooker, Foster, Banner, Payne, & Jackson, 1998; Lintern, Woods, & Phair, 2000b). It has been used extensively for this purpose in a wide variety of formal care settings. DCM has also been used as a focus for staff training interventions. Trainers within organizations may use DCM as a means for planning tailor-made person-centered care training and as a baseline against which to measure the effectiveness of training interventions. DCM has also been used by a variety of clinicians and professionals as part of assessment, particularly when a person with dementia communicates distress. DCM observations can shed light on what might appear to be an intractable situation and, in this way, can assist in care planning. Furthermore, DCM has been used to assess the general quality of a service by some Inspection Teams (S. Heiser, personal communication, November 2001).

Although the most frequent use of DCM has focused on practice development and its application in care settings, the majority of publications that cite DCM have used it as an outcome measure. Evaluative researchers have found DCM to be an attractive measure. Given that this group, by nature, is going to publish, its members have contributed most of the journal articles on DCM. DCM has been used as a general outcome measure of care practice (Ballard, Fossey, et al., 2001; Ballard, O'Brien, et al., 2001; Innes & Surr, 2001). It also has been used to evaluate the effects of therapeutic intervention (Brooker, 2001; Brooker & Duce, 2000) or changes in care practice, especially around relocation (Kitwood, Buckland, & Petre, 1995) and staff training (Lintern, Woods, & Phair, 2000a). DCM was not intended to be used primarily as a research measure. In the absence of other viable measures of well-being, however, particularly in the 1990s, DCM has been used as an outcome measure and has yielded some interesting results. More specific research measures have since been developed. As of 2002, a body of research is being undertaken to determine whether DCM stands as a valid research instrument compared with these other measures. There is also research being undertaken to assess the reliability of DCM in a much more rigorous manner than in the past.

In the future, DCM will probably become a set of related methods that can be used for different purposes. The family of DCM measures could consist of

1. An improved version that provides rich data for developmental evaluations and care-planning purposes

2. A research outcome measure that separates quality of life and quality of care measures

3. A short version that can be used for inspection and benchmark purposes

The challenge will be whether DCM can maintain a coherent structure and still be fit for these purposes.

DEFINING THE SETTING CONDITIONS FOR IMPROVING PRACTICE WITH DEMENTIA CARE MAPPING

Any tool is only as good as the skills of the person using it. DCM is a powerful tool that can be used poorly; in some instances, it damages the self-esteem of staff. In turn, this has a negative effect on the people with dementia for whom these staff provide care. When DCM is used as part of an overall quality strategy with practice development at its heart, the tool can achieve the following (Brooker & Rogers, 2001):

*   Reduce levels of ill-being and increase levels of well-being

*   Provide both quantitative and qualitative data about increased well-being

*   Reduce or eradicate staff-generated examples of malignant social psychology

*   Refocus care to the most dependent residents within a dementia care setting (as a result of progressive cycles of quality improvement that target the care plans of individuals who have poor levels of well-being)

*   Provide a shared language and focus across professional disciplines, caregiving staff, and management teams

*   Be considered a valid measure by direct care staff as well as those responsible for managing and commissioning care

*   Improve the care practice of staff trained in DCM

*   Improve job satisfaction, which can decrease staff turnover

DCM needs to be embedded within an overall positive management framework that emphasizes practice development (Cox, 2001). DCM does not exist in a vacuum. Those with experience using DCM (e.g., Bolton et al., 2000) cite reflective practice, a shared value base, supervision, training in person-centered care, and staff development as preconditions for DCM. At the beginning of the 21st century, the challenge to researchers and practitioners is to identify the minimum and necessary setting conditions for DCM to achieve a positive outcome.

One issue that has also attracted attention is the characteristics of people within care organizations who have taken DCM forward. DCM leaders in successful DCM projects apparently have sufficient authority to allocate resources or have the backing to do so. They also can organize DCM implementation, troubleshoot, and ensure that feedback is used. They are able to communicate at all levels of the organization, usually have a considerable knowledge of dementia care and therapy, are well organized, and are able to produce reports quickly and accurately.

The interaction of the process of DCM with individuals and organizational structures is complex and requires much unraveling. The challenge will be whether it is possible to unravel the complex steps without falling flat on our faces.

THE EIGHTH EDITION OF THE DEMENTIA CARE MAPPING TRAINING MANUAL

The current edition of the DCM training manual was launched in 1997 at an event called "DCM: The Next Five Years." Kitwood, of the Bradford Dementia Group, led the event and apparently thought that this seventh edition (Bradford Dementia Group, 1997) would be good until 2002. Certainly, in 2002, consensus exists for change on a number of issues. Numerous research projects are underway that will help the Bradford Dementia Group base the eighth edition on empirical data. Given the outcome of these projects, as well as field-testing and development time, 2004 is a realistic launch date for the eighth edition of the DCM manual.

Two main criticisms from practitioners about DCM are the length of time that it takes and its complexity. Research will demonstrate how simpler measures correlate with DCM and the added value of conducting a full DCM evaluation (Brooker, 1999). Empirical data can also determine the necessary time period for conducting valid maps and whether continuous observation is necessary in all contexts. The challenge is to make the measures simpler without making them superficial or unfit for their purposes. This chapter has already alluded to the fact that a number of tools will likely be fit for different purposes. Simpler measures may be just as effective in some situations. In addition, some coding anomalies within the current edition could be simplified, although some codes might require expansion.

Related to complexity is the issue of reliability. In research studies, a concordance reliability coefficient of 0.8 appears achievable for interrater reliability and across time; however, this level is much more variable in ordinary evaluation maps. Given the complexity of the method, drift is likely to occur among different trainers and different projects. The challenge is to build mechanisms that increase reliability in routine maps. The equality of training experiences and a standard, detailed manual are the main ways of achieving this as of 2002. In the future, it may be possible to post video scenarios on the Internet every few months, which all mappers need to code correctly (or against a gold standard) to maintain their accreditation. Standardized Internet training in the basic DCM method is another means by which reliability of training experience could be ensured.

Standardized computerized data collection and analysis and report writing are long overdue. Many mappers have developed their own programs for data analysis. The possibility of including standard software in the basic course is being investigated, and this will certainly be part of the eighth edition.

Another challenge is developing a tool that can be used as an adjunct to DCM in private areas of the care setting or in people's homes. Well and Illbeing Profiling (Bruce, 2000) is a useful addition for this endeavor. Also, research is underway in people's homes, where a mapper memorizes and uses the codes as a basis for notes following his or her intervention (Carr & Coleman, 2001).

The DCM evaluation should include comments from people with dementia who are able to say how they feel about the care process. In the early 21st century, the voice of the person with dementia is considered important and needs to be heard directly whenever possible. DCM was an early attempt to put the perspective of the person with dementia into a pluralistic evaluative framework. There are clear examples in which the direct voice of people with dementia and DCM have been used as complementary parts of a pluralistic evaluation (Barnett, 2000). DCM is not an alternative to hearing the direct voice; rather, it offers a complementary viewpoint. Providing direct feedback about services on which one totally depends for health and well-being means that some people report being satisfied with even poor service quality (Brooker, 1997). The relationship between these two viewpoints will no doubt receive greater emphasis within the eighth edition of the DCM manual.

A positive person work coding frame needs to be developed, expanding on the descriptions in *Dementia Reconsidered: The Person Comes First* (Kitwood, 1997). The current DCM manual's Positive Event Record does not have the same status or clear link to theory as the Personal Detraction coding. Many practitioners are experimenting with ways to incorporate a record of positive person work within the current DCM tool, and such concepts are now taught in basic DCM training. The challenge is how to fully incorporate these ideas into the eighth edition without making the tool even more unwieldy and complex.

CONCLUSION

The Think Tank 2001 event was the first time that a significant number of DCM stakeholders gathered since the launch of the manual's seventh edition in 1997. In her closing speech, Downs, the head of Bradford Dementia Group, emphasized the need for the DCM community to meet more frequently and for networks to develop around specific interests. DCM appears to touch something universal within those involved in person-centered care—across disciplines, across professional backgrounds, across language barriers, and across cultures. By their nature, practitioners who are passionate about dementia care are also passionate about communication and usually want to share their experiences with others. They tend to be busy people, however, and there is a future challenge for Bradford Dementia Group to provide mappers with easily accessible resources to ensure best use of the tool. There is a saying in the quality assurance field along the lines of "make it easy for people to get it right the first time." The challenge is harnessing this energy in a network for improving the quality of care for people with dementia everywhere and providing backup and resources that make it as easy as possible, both practically and emotionally, to be a Dementia Care Mapper.

REFERENCES

Ballard, C., Fossey, J., Chithramohan, R., Howard, R., Burns, A., Thompson, P., Tadros, G., & Fairbairn, A. (2001). Quality of care in private sector and NHS facilities for people with dementia: Cross sectional survey. *British Medical Journal, 323,* 426–427.

Ballard, C., O'Brien, J., James, I., Mynt, P., Lana, M., Potkins, D., Reichelt, K., Lee, L., Swann, A., & Fossey, J. (2001). Quality of life for people with dementia living in residential and nursing home care: The impact of performance on activities of daily living, behavioral and psychological symptoms, language skills, and psychotropic drugs. *International Psychogeriatrics, 13*(1), 93–106.

Barnett, E. (2000). *Including the person with dementia in designing and delivering care: 'I need to be me!'* London: Jessica Kingsley Publishers.

Bolton, J., Gee, I., Jackson, L., Mather, D., Potter, L., Roberts, S., Robson, P., Scurfield, M., Stewart, D., & Vandor, C. (2000). Stepping back to move forward with DCM. *Journal of Dementia Care, 8*(4), 26–28.

Bradford Dementia Group. (1997). *Evaluating dementia care: The DCM method* (7th ed.). Bradford, England: University of Bradford.

Brooker, D. (1997). Issues in user feedback on health services for elderly people. *British Journal of Nursing, 6,* 159–162.

Brooker, D. (1999). DCM and engagement combined to audit care quality. *The Journal of Dementia Care, 7*(3), 33–36.

Brooker, D. (2001). Enriching lives: evaluation of the ExtraCare Activity Challenge. *Journal of Dementia Care, 9*(3), 33–37.

Brooker, D., & Duce, L. (2000). Wellbeing and activity in dementia: a comparison of group reminiscence therapy, structured goal-directed group activity and unstructured time. *Ageing & Mental Health, 4*(4), 354–358.

Brooker, D., Foster, N., Banner, A., Payne, M., & Jackson, L. (1998). The efficacy of Dementia Care Mapping as an audit tool: Report of a 3-year British NHS evaluation. *Ageing & Mental Health, 2*(1), 60–70.

Brooker, D., & Rogers, L. (Eds.). (2001). *DCM think tank transcripts 2001.* Bradford, England: University of Bradford.

Bruce, E. (2000). Looking after well-being: A tool for evaluation. *Journal of Dementia Care, 8*(6), 25–27.

Carr, A., & Coleman, P. (2001, August). Methodological problems in studying the day to day lives of people with dementia. *Proceedings of the British Society of Gerontology Annual Conference.*

Cox, S. (2001). Developing quality in services. In C. Cantley (Ed.), *A handbook of dementia care* (pp. 258–277). Buckingham, England: Open University Press

Innes, A., Capstick, A., & Surr, C. (2000). Mapping out the framework. *Journal of Dementia Care, 8*(2), 20–21.

Innes, A., & Surr, C. (2001). Measuring the well-being of people with dementia living in formal care settings: The use of Dementia Care Mapping. *Aging & Mental Health, 5*(3), 258–268.

Kitwood, T. (1997). *Dementia reconsidered: The person comes first.* Buckingham, England: Open University Press.

Kitwood, T., Buckland, S., & Petre, T. (1995). *Brighter futures: A report on research into provision for persons with dementia in residential homes, nursing homes and sheltered housing.* Kidlington, England: Anchor Housing Association.

Lintern, T., Woods, R., & Phair, L. (2000a). Before and after training: A case study of intervention. *Journal of Dementia Care, 8*(1), 15–17.

Lintern, T., Woods, R., & Phair, L. (2000b). Training is not enough to change care practice. *Journal of Dementia Care, 8*(2), 15–17.

CONCLUSION

ANTHEA INNES

Dementia Care Mapping (DCM) is at an exciting crossroads. As noted throughout this book, DCM is a tool that has only been recently accepted within the United Kingdom as a measure of well-being for individuals with dementia (Audit Commission, 2000). As is often the case when a tool gains widespread popularity, others begin to question its value. Contemporary discussions (Bolton et al., 2000; Brooker, 2000; Dewing, 2000) suggest DCM's weaknesses, such as the coding frames' psychometric basis and the partial view of care that DCM provides. The contributors to this book add to the debate by making many interesting comments on the method, its strengths, its limitations, and—crucially—how these limitations can be addressed within the cultural context in which the method operates. The Bradford Dementia Group has plans for a new version of the DCM manual (Chapter 11). With the eighth edition of the manual, then, there is an opportunity to address directly the problematic aspects of the method that have been raised throughout this book (Chapters 1 and 4 in particular).

One such weakness is "the mechanics" of the method. The coding frames on which DCM relies are based on a subjective decision (albeit informed by empirical study), which is problematic if one approaches the issue from a quasi-positivistic worldview (i.e., a research and evaluation standpoint that views the world as a science laboratory where cause and effect can be determined; of course, a care setting cannot be controlled in the way that a scientific experiment can). Yet, perhaps the value of DCM's coding frames is their grounding

155

in the philosophy of person-centered care, with the aim of evaluating the extent to which person-centered care is a reality for people receiving care.

Any coding frame is open to question, as all are initially based on subjective views and then packaged as objective measures. This may be a weakness of DCM, which claims to encapsulate quantitative and qualitative analysis, although attempts could be made to produce reliable and valid coding frames within a paradigm that is concerned with objective, reliable, and valid measures (Chapter 2). The seventh edition of the DCM manual (Bradford Dementia Group, 1997) outlines a descriptive quantitative analysis that those using the method can compute with relative ease. Confusion about the value of such basic analyses arises when individuals attempt to apply complex statistical tests, such as parametric tests, to data that is not fully amenable to such an approach (e.g., a methodological position taken in an interpretivist school of thought [Goffman, 1967; Layder, 1994], the ethnological stance outlined in the DCM manual). It would perhaps be more fruitful to explore further the qualitative data that DCM engenders. Linking this qualitative data to the social world may be a positive move forward for DCM. It may create opportunities to explore structural issues that threaten the delivery of quality person-centered care (Chapter 9).

Challenges remain, however, when one moves beyond discussions about the mechanics or operationalization of the coding frames. As pointed out in Chapter 1, the theoretical basis of DCM is often overlooked. In turn, this can lead to a lack of interest in developing the method's theory but a wealth of interest in its mechanics. Clearly the latter is important. Yet, can the method truly evolve and develop if theoretical underpinnings are not questioned, reexamined, and developed to account for the ever-increasing interest in dementia and dementia care, the setting of quality care standards, and the inclusion of the voices of individuals with dementia in the debates on care and varying perspectives about dementia—be they biomedical, psychological, or social perspectives?

It is acknowledged throughout this book that one of DCM's powerful contributions is the popularization of person-centered care but that change and development of care practices can perhaps be better achieved by other means, such as practice development (Chapters 4 and 5) and staff development (Chapter 6). It is of interest that the person-centered approach to care is a topic of controversy and debate (Packer, 2000), with care practitioners questioning whether person-centered care can ever be a reality (Packer, 2000; Poole, 2000). These discussions appear to eschew the necessary understanding of the interface between care practice and cultural change. Fundamental to the apparent lack of insight into this process is the fragmentation of care provision from historical, social, political, and economic systems. A central flaw of the initial grumblings about DCM is the apparent misconception that DCM in and of itself can be a route to achieving cultural change and person-centered care. As contributors have noted throughout this book (Chapters 3, 4, 6, 7, 8, 9, and 10), other issues require consideration: the culture of the care setting, the social context, individual cultural factors, and organizational cultural factors. DCM is a method, a means to evaluate care provision at a particular moment in time in a particular place. Clearly, it cannot be a change agent, as many would naïvely—if optimistically—hope. Therefore, DCM's value is its ability to evaluate care by looking at the subjective experiences of life in a care setting. It is not a tool that can achieve change in and of itself. Those using the method may find that the process of conducting observations, analyzing data, and sharing both with staff highlights areas that need attention, but the method itself is not designed to address such issues. It is crucial that people who consider using DCM—both care providers and researchers—understand that evaluating care from the DCM perspective will not change care provision, nor will it produce the hard data of the positivist research paradigm. DCM is an observation method, providing a framework for viewing care practices and subjectively assigning a numerical value to what is observed (i.e., a qualitative code that is numerically defined). The data may raise awareness among those providing care, but raising an individual's awareness of a subject does not guarantee a change in that person's behavior. Thus, as of 2002, the value of DCM is evident in the following:

1. Its ability to raise staff's awareness of their collective care practices if the mapper adheres to the DCM process, although this does not necessarily lead to change (Chapter 6)

2. The observation schema that enables researchers and practitioners to observe care in a semistructured framework

3. The possibility of linking observed practices with the person-centered care philosophy

DCM data can provide a framework to document the care experience of a resident group and of many individuals over time. The data can be used to develop care plans for people with dementia (Chapter 5) and to identify staff development issues (Chapter 6). Thus, DCM may lead to certain outcomes, depending on the user's ability to influence practice and the organization's willingness to support the required changes (Chapter 7). DCM's undeveloped potential lies primarily in the possibility of linking observable microlevel practices not only to the theory of person-centered care, but also to wider influences on care practices and implementing the theory in systems that are not initially conducive to person-centered care.

Two key unresolved problems have been created by using the method for purposes that it was not intended to address. First, if DCM is used as a research instrument within the traditional research paradigm (commonly known as *positivism*), how can one create a reliable and valid tool? That is, not an ecologically valid tool but a scientific tool that is reliable and valid (Chapter 2). Second, DCM is ethically opposed to viewing private portions of the care setting (e.g., bathrooms). Can users who want to observe the entire care setting use DCM without breaching its ethical principles? Although some may purport to attaining a global view, it is worth bearing in mind that no care setting can ever be viewed in its entirety—the observer's views, the utilized tools, and the data analysis produce a partial view of the setting under scrutiny.

There are doubtless several other problems that could be stated and debated; however, one must return to the issue of purpose—what does DCM claim to do? What does the user (either a researcher or care provider) hope to achieve? Is DCM the appropriate tool to help achieve that purpose? It could be argued that using DCM in a cultural context that is designed to "manage" behaviors (Chapter 8) constitutes misuse, as the philosophy on which DCM is based seeks to understand rather than to manage behaviors. Yet, Chapter 8 illustrates that the method has been successfully used and indeed embraced by a culture that may initially appear to contradict DCM's ethos.

This book's contributors believe that DCM's value lies in its contribution to changing the culture of dementia care—not just in the United Kingdom, where DCM was born, but around the world, where innovative individuals and organizations (Chapters 4, 7, 8, and 9) have embraced Kitwood's (1997) philosophy and the opportunity to evaluate the extent to which care is person centered at points in time. DCM may lead to certain outcomes (Chapters 3, 5, 6, and 7), but this depends on the user and the agency or the action exercised by individuals and the collective group (throughout the organization). That it offers the individual this possibility is perhaps its greatest attraction—and also its downfall if those using and promoting the method do not make this point explicit.

Even if such questions are considered, policy will be lacking until all who are involved in dementia care (practitioners, researchers, and policy makers) actively seek and listen to the voices of those providing and receiving care on a daily basis. It will be based on misconceptions about the state of dependency that is enforced by placing older people with dementia in institutions, thereby excluding them from society. A more radical reform of care provision is necessary, addressing the physical location of care settings; the social, economic, and political position of those providing care; and the position of care recipients.

Policy makers must also account for wider social, political, and economic factors (Innes, 2002). The low social and economic status awarded to staff who care for older people urgently needs to be addressed if care for people with dementia is to improve. The history of undervaluing care work (synonymous with "women's work"), older people, and people with dementia must be fully explored if policy makers are to influence and improve care provision for people with dementia and conditions for paid caregivers. DCM is one tool to draw on for change.

REFERENCES

Audit Commission. (2000). *Forget me not: Mental health services for older people.* London: Author.

Bolton, J., Gee, I., Jackson, L., Mather, D., Potter, L., Roberts, S., Robson, P., Scurfield, M., Stewart, D., & Vandor, C. (2000). Stepping back to move forward with DCM. *Journal of Dementia Care, 8*(4), 26–28.

Bradford Dementia Group. (1997). *Evaluating dementia care: The DCM method* (7th ed.). Bradford, England: University of Bradford.

Brooker, D.J.R. (2000). Dementia Care Mapping: How is it being used in 2000? In A. Dickinson, H. Bartlett, & S. Wade (Eds.), *Old Age in a New Age: Proceedings of the British Society of Gerontology 29th Annual Conference* (pp. 15–19). Oxford, England: Oxford Brookes University Press.

Dewing, J. (2000, September). *DCM, methodological issues and practice development.* Paper presented at Old Age in a New Age: British Society of Gerontology 29th Annual Conference, Oxford, England.

Goffman, E. (1967). *Interaction ritual.* London: Anchor Books.

Innes, A. (2002). The social and political context of formal dementia care provision. *Ageing and Society, 22*(4).

Kitwood, T. (1997). *Dementia reconsidered: The person comes first.* Buckingham, England: Open University Press.

Layder, D.R. (1994). *Understanding social theory.* Thousand Oaks, CA: Sage Publications.

Packer, T. (2000). Does person-centred care exist? *Journal of Dementia Care, 8*(3), 19–21.

Poole, J. (2000). Person-centred care: Across the bridge from ideal to reality. *Journal of Dementia Care, 8*(4), 8–9.

INDEX

Page references followed by *t* or *f* indicate tables or figures, respectively.